Ritual Healing in the Zion Christian Church in South Africa

Bloomsbury Studies in Black Religion and Cultures

Series Editors: Anthony B. Pinn and Monica R. Miller

Bloomsbury Studies in Black Religion and Cultures advances innovative scholarship that reimagines and animates the global study of Black religions, culture and identity across space and time. The series publishes scholarship that addresses the mutually constitutive nature of race and religion and the social, cultural, intellectual and material effects of religio-racial formations and identities. The series welcomes projects that address and foreground the intersectional and constitutive nature of Black religions and cultures and privileges work that is inter/transdisciplinary and methodologically intersectional in nature.

African Spirituality, Politics and Knowledge Systems
Toyin Falola
Black Transhuman Liberation Theology
Philip Butler
Innovation and Competition in Zimbabwean Pentecostalism
Edited by Ezra Chitando
Speculations on Black Life
Edited by Darrell Jones, Monifa Love and Anthony Pinn
Religion and Inequality in Africa
Edited by Ezra Chitando, Loreen Maseno and Joram Tarusarira
Decolonizing Contemporary Gospel Music through Praxis
Robert Beckford
Ben Ammi Ben Israel
Michael T. Miller
Inventing the New Dispensation in Zimbabwe
Edited by Ezra Chitando, Lovemore Togarasei and Joram Tarusarira

Ritual Healing in the Zion Christian Church in South Africa

Mookgo Solomon Kgatle

BLOOMSBURY ACADEMIC
LONDON • NEW YORK • OXFORD • NEW DELHI • SYDNEY

BLOOMSBURY ACADEMIC
Bloomsbury Publishing Plc, 50 Bedford Square, London, WC1B 3DP, UK
Bloomsbury Publishing Inc, 1385 Broadway, New York, NY 10018, USA
Bloomsbury Publishing Ireland, 29 Earlsfort Terrace, Dublin 2, D02 AY28, Ireland

BLOOMSBURY, BLOOMSBURY ACADEMIC and the Diana logo are trademarks of Bloomsbury Publishing Plc

First published in Great Britain 2026

Series design by Maria Rajka
Cover image © Brooks Kraft / Getty Images

A catalogue record for this book is available from the British Library.

A catalogue record for this book is available from the Library of Congress.

ISBN: HB: 978-1-3505-5287-6
ePDF: 978-1-3505-5288-3
eBook: 978-1-3505-5289-0

Series: Bloomsbury Studies in Black Religion and Cultures

Typeset by Newgen KnowledgeWorks Pvt. Ltd., Chennai, India

For product safety related questions contact productsafety@bloomsbury.com.

To find out more about our authors and books visit www.bloomsbury.com and sign up for our newsletters.

Contents

Preface

I grew up in the Zion Christian Church where my father also served as a minister and the rest of the family as members. My grandfather was also a staunch member and minister of the church for years. Therefore, for me, the Zion Christian Church can be considered a family church because all my uncles and aunts are still members. What fascinated me was how the church approached the concept of healing as opposed to other Christian churches. While other Christian churches used the conventional laying on of hands when praying for the sick, my father and other ministers in the Zion Christian Church would use different symbols, ceremonies and other rituals to acquire healing for the sick. This kind of healing is called ritual healing in this book. The argument is that the ritual healing process in the Zion Christian Church should be distinguished from the traditional African medicine. For example, I can confirm that I have never consulted a sangoma, an Inyanga or even a diviner for healing while being a member of the Zion Christian Church. Therefore, the association of the ritual healing process in the Zion Christian Church with traditional African medicine is very unfortunate.

In the Zion Christian Church, I was mainly fascinated by how worship was conducted, given that worship, in my view, formed part of the healing process in the church. My father was not just a minister of the word in the Zion Christian Church but was also a singer in his own right, and he would continuously point out that he was not just singing but praying through a song. That is when I learned that music in the Zion Christian Church is part of the healing rituals of the church. Similarly, in the Zion Christian Church, we would dance in the open air while it was raining – this was done in the name of prayer and as a quest to seek healing. I was also part of the male choir of the Zion Christian Church branch in my village and would dance on Friday nights and occasionally on Saturday nights as part of the church ceremony, *mpoho*. It is also true that in traditional African medicine, singing and dancing form part of the healing process. But again, the practices therefore are not the same. There is a distinction between traditional night dancing and worship nights in the Zion Christian Church. While traditional night dancing seeks to appease the spiritual world, we believed that singing and dancing in the night were part of spiritual warfare against witchcraft and other spiritual forces in the spiritual world. Thus, in engaging in such night prayers, as the believers in the Zion Christian Church, we engaged in spiritual warfare.

My father, as a minister of the Zion Christian Church, would sprinkle water around the house to bring protection against witchcraft and other forms of spiritual attack. This too was different from the traditional African medicine practices as sprinkling of water is done to confront the very evil spirits existing in the spirit realm espoused by traditional religions in Africa. In the Zion Christian Church and our house, there were extra measures that were taken for the protection of the family but this should not be linked with traditional African medicine protective measures. The only challenge was that my father would sprinkle water on my school books, which I would later struggle to use because of the water. My father would explain that this was done to protect my books against witchcraft at the school as well as jealousy on the part of other learners. Therefore, spiritual protection against witchcraft, sorcery and other forms of spiritual attacks was done using objects and symbols that must be separated from traditional African medicine.

As a young man in the Zion Christian Church, I was always intrigued by men or even women who would come and pick up others to speak privately with them outside the church. It was also a practice during the normal Sunday service for someone to rise and point to another believer to address them. This was later explained to me as the practice of prophecy within the church where the challenges that people are going through in life are revealed through a word of prophecy. I did not see anything wrong with this practice as a young person in the church. I was always attracted by how many prophets in our branch church would enter some sort of trance when they were about to deliver a prophecy. Others would shout and speak strangely in other tongues, some of them making sounds. I was also surprised that only the elderly would qualify as the recipients of the prophecies, and it was my strong wish to also be pointed out to receive prophecy. The practices of prophecy are common within other African Independent Churches. However, they are not necessarily linked with traditional African medicine practices such as divination. This will be explained later in the book.

Growing up in a poor family where basic needs such as food were not given, I wondered why it was that the family was not allowed to eat certain foods such as Mopani worms which can be picked from a tree. I was also surprised that we were not allowed to eat pork, which was also affordable at that time compared to other meat such as beef, lamb and goat meat. I later understood that there are church-related taboos and restrictions when it comes to what is permissible to eat and what is not. Therefore, I had enriched experiences in the Zion Christian Church concerning healing, prophecy, worship and even social restrictions. However, this book is more than just my recollections of what I used to experience in the Zion Christian Church, leaning as it does towards a scholarly reflection on the ritual healing process in the church. However, my experiences as shared above will enrich the discussions in this book as I was part of the church for many years (14 to be precise).

Mookgo Solomon Kgatle
Pretoria, South Africa

1

Introduction

Ritual healing process: Framing the discourse

Ritual healing is a therapeutic process that uses symbolic actions, ceremonies and healing rituals to help improve the mental, physical or social well-being of individuals (Csordas 1983:2). The ritual healing process is used in the studies linked to anthropology, particularly religious studies, performance arts, cultural studies and therapy (Csordas 1999; Mclenon 2004; Stephenson 2015). McClenon (2004:121) adds: 'Ritual healing theory hypotheses are testable within the domains of psychical research, anthropology, archaeology, social psychology of religion, folklore, history, physiology, and medicine.' Archaeologically, it can be argued that ritual healing was part of human existence in the past (Stephenson 2015:1). This framework has been used mainly in anthropological studies to assess patients' healing process through various rituals in the human body. The word 'Ritual' has a human element, particularly in the use of symbols and objects by humanity in general, even before we can speak of healing or its application in religion (Stephenson 2015:1). Ritual healing is part of human nature and human socialization, sociality, culture and customs. According to Stephenson (2015:1), each human being – whether or not religious – has somehow been part of ritual healing in their lives as they participate in important ceremonies such as weddings, funerals, parades, liturgies, exchange of gifts and unveiling of tombstones. These rites and ritual ceremonies have crossed one's life at some point even if one is not religiously inclined. Therefore, it can be reiterated that the practice of ritual healing has been part of human life for a long time. The same can be said of the African context, where ritual healing has been part of African cosmology such that ritual healing has become widely accepted even outside the religious spectrum. Therefore, according to Field (2022:121), ritual healing is based on 'ancient knowledge that produces beneficial action for all beings on the planet. It centers ritual voices and definitions of healing, emphasizing land, relationships, and spiritual connections.' This means that ritual healing can be used as per the determination of a specific religious group because its original foundation is not necessarily religious. Hence, I argue in this book that both traditional African religions and African Independent Churches have different approaches to ritual healing.

Ritual healing is very popular in the African context, such that even during the Covid-19 pandemic, many Africans survived by using ritual healing; some could not use biomedical treatment, and others resisted vaccinations. Among those who resisted vaccinations were members of the African Independent Churches such as the Zion Christian Church and other churches (Humbe 2023:204). This was not the first time that these churches shunned Western or modern medicine and embraced ritual healing to deal with the challenges of sickness and diseases. In this case, ritual healing became a popular practice in dealing with the challenges of Covid-19. Ritual healing is not only seen in the context of religious practices, as highlighted above, but also in the use of self-medication. During the Covid-19 pandemic, the author observed that most Black people in South Africa used self-medication to deal with the virus. This means that modern medicine is not the only way in which African people deal with the challenges of diseases; ritual healing is an alternative. Although the focus of this book is not Covid-19, the point made here is that ritual healing is very popular among the African Independent Churches, to the extent that it became an option even during a pandemic such as Covid-19. In addition, it is to point out that even outside religious practices, ritual healing became popular among many Africans who mixed concoctions to resist the virus. Therefore, it is not always correct that the use of ritual healing represents a syncretistic nature in the Zion Christian Church and other African Independent Churches.

Ritual healing should therefore be considered to be very different from orthodox practices of healing such as the use of Western medicine and psychiatric treatment. The ritual healing theory is relevant in tracing the origin of healing practices within a specific religious group. It is important in the theorization of healing rituals in a religious group such as the Zion Christian Church (McGuire & Kantor 1988). This theory is useful in arguing that the various rituals used for the healing of individuals can result in physiological healing within the religious group. Hence, ritual healing is not only defined in terms of spiritual healing but rather as holistic healing that includes the emotional, physical and spiritual aspects of the human being. Ritual healing is used within social anthropology and other humanities as a theory that is relevant to overturning the existing condition of patients and their challenges of sicknesses and diseases.

Ritual healing is performative, using various objects and symbols, and applying them in the process of healing for those suffering from sicknesses and diseases (Steinbock 1982:181). Hence, in the African context, as discussed above, it is applied through rites, ceremonies and festivals to deal with diseases among patients. These aspects of the ritual healing process are discussed and applied to the Zion Christian Church in the rest of the book. The aim of using the ritual healing process is to demonstrate that the healing rituals in the Zion Christian Church differ from traditional African medicine.

Ritual healing process in African Independent Churches

The ritual healing process in Zion Christian Church in South Africa is premised here on the broader framework of the ritual healing process within the African Independent Churches (AICs) as this church is widely categorized in the latter. The abbreviation AICs can refer to African Initiated Churches, African Instituted Churches, African Indigenous Churches and African Independent Churches. My preference is for the term 'African Independent Churches', and to avoid confusion, I do not use the abbreviation in this book. One of the reasons I use African Independent Churches is that these churches exist because of the need to become independent from the Western missionary churches that were aligned to the racial oppression at that time, particularly in the South African context. Thus, African Independent Churches are churches that focus on becoming relevant to the African context by practising church activities without following the Western epistemological systems. However, this should not be grounds for always perceiving the African Independent Churches as breakaway churches as there are many African Independent Churches that do not have prior connections with the Western missionary churches. There are different types of African Independent Churches in the South African context and elsewhere on the continent, such as messianic churches, Ethiopian-type churches, Aladura churches and Spirit-type churches. The messianic African Independent Churches are known for their adoration of and dependence on their leader who, in a way, is respected in the same way as the person Jesus Christ is and becomes the messiah of their followers – a kind of 'Black Jesus', so to speak (Oosthuizen 1992; Anderson 1999; Daneel 2000). The idea of a 'Black Jesus' sells in the African context as some believe it liberates them from colonialism, which they confuse with Western forms of Christianity. One such example is the Nazareth Baptist Church of Isaiah Shembe in KwaZulu-Natal whose emphasis on the leader has contributed to the church being known as the 'Shembe church' and its followers as the 'adherents of Shembe' (Kumalo & Mujinga 2017:123). The Ethiopian-type African Independent Churches emphasize their foundations on the African continent and that the churches in Africa should be led by Black people (Oosthuizen 2000). The Aladura African Independent Churches are found mainly in the Nigerian context and are known for their emphasis on prayer, for referring to the baptism in the Holy Spirit and for showing evidence of speaking in tongues (Anderson 1991). They include Nigerian churches, such as the Christ Apostolic Church, the Cherubim and Seraphim movement, the Celestial Church of Christ and the Church of the Lord (Adogame 2000; Adedibu, Akindolie & Olujobi 2022).

The Zion Christian Church might be considered a spirit-type African Independent Church (Anderson 1991). As highlighted above, to understand the ritual healing process in the Zion Christian Church, there is a need to understand it in African Independent Churches. The ritual healing process in traditional African religions has been explored in the past, particularly concerning the use of indigenous knowledge systems in the healing of Africans. However, the ritual healing process in the African Independent Churches requires more reflection. Daneel (2019) mentions the ritual healing process as one of the core practices of spirituality within the African Independent Churches. For Daneel (2019), ritual healing is one of the aspects that can draw numbers into these churches, as many in Africa are going through sicknesses and diseases and have limited access to health facilities. It is the aspect of ritual healing that has been able to draw people from the Western mission churches to the African Independent Churches. Therefore, ritual healing can be considered an integral part of the spirituality within African Independent Churches that has made these churches attractive to Africans. Hence, those who are healed are asked to testify to make ritual healing popular among the people. According to Daneel (2019:16), the African Independent Churches emulate the ministry of Jesus as it dealt with healing as many suggest that Jesus's ministry would not have flourished in the way it did without the application of healing. The African Independent Churches believe that healing is one of the central points that made Jesus's ministry popular among the people. Hence, they also emphasize healing by following the steps of Jesus Christ. Therefore, it can be concluded that healing is a deciding factor for many people in Africa when it comes to joining the African Independent Churches.

In the African Independent Churches, the ritual healing process is studied by taking into cognizance the role of the prophets in effecting healing among the people (Daneel 2019). Most of the African Independent Churches are led by a 'prophet' figure who is perceived to be carrying special powers for the healing of the people. Some prophets in the African Independent Churches point to God as the healer so that people shift their focus away from the prophet and look up to God for healing as idolization of prophets has the potential to mistake them as diviners. However, in the minds of the people, the prophet remains the one carrying special powers for their healing. In the gospels, Jesus would always refer the people to his Father as the healer of the people to shift the focus of the people away from him, leading them to focus on God, the Father. African Independent Churches have a propensity to focus on a prophet who carries healing powers. However, I argue here that prophets in African Independent Churches should be differentiated from diviners in traditional African religions.

Most African Independent Churches use certain objects or substances, particularly water, for the healing of the people as part of the ritual healing process. Depending on the type of the African Independent Church concerned, there would also be other objects used for ritual healing. Daneel (2019) points out that the use of objects in ritual healing is very close to the practices involved in the thought processes of African Independent Churches. However, some prophets would defend the use of symbols and objects in ritual healing, arguing that they are not the source but merely symbols that signify the real power of God for the healing of the people. Daneel (2019:44) says that, for prophets in African Independent Churches, 'the objects used during [healing] are primarily the visual symbolic concretization of the Divine Power, which in itself has no medicative effect'. Therefore, when examining ritual healing in the African Independent Churches, it is important to assess the links with ritual healing in the use of plants, herbs, music and spirituality in healing. However, this link, as argued by Daneel (2019), does not always demonstrate the connection with traditional African medicine, as objects in healing are used not as a system of belief but rather as symbolic.

Ritual healing process in the Zion Christian Church

Previous studies have looked at the ritual healing process in the Zion Christian Church. One such study is the doctoral thesis of Jacqueline Martha Wouters (2014). This anthropological study is important for highlighting the various healing rituals in the Zion Christian Church but does not attempt to differentiate between traditional African medicine and ritual healing. This study which only focused on the Zion Christian Church in Marabastad in Pretoria explored the role of healing in the growth of this church.

Wouters (2014) does not in her study try to make the connections or even disconnections between ritual healing in the Zion Christian Church and traditional African medicine. This is the main contribution of the current study, that is, to dissociate ritual healing in the Zion Christian Church from traditional African medicine. Another important study is Müller (2016) which is also important for understanding the ritual of pilgrimage of the Zionist movement in South Africa. Two gaps can be identified in Müller (2016). One, it does not focus directly on ritual healing but covers the ritual of pilgrimage to a large degree. Second, it focuses on the ritual of pilgrimage as a tool to unite the fragmented social groups in the South African context but not necessarily the discussions on healing rituals. Müller (2016) remains useful in general understanding of the ritual healing process in the Zion Christian Church. Müller (2015) does make connections between the Zion Christian Church and Indigenous Christianity; however, this was not done on the theme of the ritual healing process. Therefore, this current study is relevant and contributes knowledge on the ritual healing process in the Zion Christian Church and its dissociation with traditional African medicine.

Another important work by Cabrita (2018) is opposed to the popular connections between traditional African beliefs and the Zion Christian Church by arguing that ritual healing in churches such as the Zion Christian Church should be seen as continuing a long tradition of healing in global Protestantism. Cabrita (2018) is very close to what I want to achieve in the current study. However, in my analysis, I do not link the Zion Christian Church with Global Protestantism but study the ritual healing process to dissociate it from traditional African medicine. Besides Cabrita does not delve into specific healing rituals in the Zion Christian Church in South Africa. Nonetheless, Cabrita (2018) will be one of the main sources for this current study as it helps in dissociating the ritual healing practices in the Zion Christian Church from traditional African medicine. Another important work for this study is Daneel (2019) but does not look at ritual healing in the Zion Christian Church in South Africa as I do in the current study but rather at ritual healing in Zimbabwe, the former Rhodesia. However, we cannot underestimate the common healing practices that exist between the Zion Christian Church in Zimbabwe founded by Bishop Samuel Mutendi, and the Zion Christian Church in South Africa founded by Engenas Lekganyane. Therefore as I study the ritual healing practices in the latter, I will reflect a bit on the ritual healing practices in the Zimbabwean context which by the way is very close to the South African context.

In the current study, I will also rely on the works of Allan Anderson (1999, 2000), particularly on addressing prophecy as a healing ritual in the church. The different practices of prophecy including oracular, diagnostic and prescriptive practices are discussed in the work of Anderson (1999). Anderson (1999) is also important for the biographical study of the leaders of the Zion Christian Church such as Engenas Lekganyane, Edward Lekganyane and Barnabas Lekganyane. Anderson (1999) relied much on the master dissertation of Lukhaimane (1980) which is also important for this current study. Lukhaimane's (1980) dissertation and Moripe's (1996) thesis are some of the few empirical research projects done on the Zion Christian Church. These therefore contain an important historical background of the early foundations of the Zion Christian Church. Anderson (2000) is an important book for me as a Pentecostal scholar; however, in this current study, I do not put much emphasis on the intersections of Zion and Pentecost. Anderson (2000), like many works quoted above, I must reiterate, has not specifically looked at the distinctions between traditional African medicine and the ritual healing process in the Zion Christian Church. This is the gap that the current study seeks to fill.

Therefore, this book is unique for the study of the ritual healing process in the Zion Christian Church. There are about four reasons why this study is important. Firstly, while there are scholarly books on the Zion Christian Church, the distinctions between traditional African medicine and the ritual healing process in the Zion Christian Church are yet to be explored. Secondly, we don't have a clear and definitive conceptualization of ritual healing theology within the African Independent Churches. The Zion Christian Church, as one of the largest African Independent churches, is relevant in the development of a ritual healing theology in the African Independent Churches. Thirdly, the use of healing rituals in the African Independent Churches, such as the Zion Christian Church, have been considered syncretistic by some scholars. This current study makes a unique contribution by challenging this view in assessing the whole ritual healing process in the Zion Christian Church in South Africa. Fourthly, the Zion Christian Church is one of the churches where various healing practices, as well as the practices of prophecy, worship, spiritual protection and social restrictions, can be contrasted with traditional African medicine. Therefore, this church is relevant in the study of the ritual healing process in African Independent Churches using these various practices. All of these themes will be discussed to delink traditional African medicine with the ritual healing process in the Zion Christian Church in South Africa.

Distinctions with traditional African medicine

Traditional African medicine refers to the use of indigenous herbs within African spirituality by traditional practitioners such as traditional healers, herbalists, shrine priests and diviners to bring healing to patients (Mokgobi 2014; Asamoah-Gyadu 2014; White 2015; Ozioma & Chinwe 2019). It is believed that traditional African medicine can heal various diseases. Traditional African medicine has been popular, particularly before the arrival of modern medicine in Africa, and is still popular even in post-colonial Africa. Ozioma and Chinwe (2019) did a study in countries such as Ghana, Tanzania, South Africa and Nigeria and found that the practice is popular in these countries. In the South African context where the majority of Black people do not have medical aid, traditional African medicine has been popularized by young and vibrant traditional practitioners who post their skills and practices on social media platforms. This has attracted other young initiates who would train as diviners, traditional healers and herbalists. Another reason for the popularity of traditional African medicine is that traditional practitioners can diagnose the spiritual cause of the disease using various mediums in African spirituality including invoking the ancestral spirits. Hence, White (2015:6) explains that doctors can refer patients to traditional practitioners if the root cause of the problem is spiritual. Therefore, traditional African medicine has in a way become an alternative to other forms of medicine not only in Africa but also elsewhere in the world. Similar to modern medicine, the diagnosis of the disease follows the prescription. The traditional practitioners can prescribe the relevant treatment to the patient which includes among others various ceremonies, rituals and herbs that the patient needs to use for the remedy.

Many scholars such as Sundkler (1961), Hanekom (1975) and Mokgobi (2014) have linked traditional African medicine with healing in African Independent Churches. To a certain extent, even scholars such as Daneel (2019) have drawn some parallelism between traditional African medicine and healing in African Independent Churches. Mokgobi (2014:1) points out that 'the traditional African philosophy of illness in most cases encompasses relations between God, ancestors and the universe; and in many traditional healers double as religious leaders (priests and prophets) in African independent churches'. In this way, Mokgobi (2014) does not make a distinction between a diviner in traditional African medicine and a prophet in African Independent Churches. One of the reasons for linking traditional African medicine and healing in African

Independent is because both use ritual healing including symbols, ceremonies and other healing rituals. In a way, they both relate to African cosmology, beliefs, customs and cultures. However, I argue that they differ in how they approach these healing rituals. The second reason is that both differ from modern scientific medicine in the ability to trace the origin of sickness not only to its physiological and psychological causes but to the spiritual and social disorders as well. Van den Bosch-Heij (2013:121) explains this relationship in this way:

> In the traditional African religious frame as well as in the religious frame of the [African Independent Churches], the existence of evil is attributed to powerful spiritual forces, who influence and control all aspects of human life. In everyday life, one has to reckon with ancestor spirits, and malevolent forces or demons, who have their agenda and who aim to undermine human well-being. Illness, misfortune, and suffering are interpreted as interventions of the spiritual realm indicating that there is a specific reason for the lack of well-being and health.

Cabrita (2018:143) concurs that 'both divine healing and African diagnosticians of this period were willing to view sickness and health not merely as physiological matters, but as profoundly spiritual conditions". In simple terms, both traditional African religions and the African Independent Churches trace the cause of sickness and diseases to the spirit realm where evil forces of darkness exist. The link is also due to the ability of both methods to provide spiritual, physical, emotional and psychological healing – meaning their ability to be holistic.

Cabrita (2018:5) points out decolonization as one of the reasons scholars jumped to conclude that African Independent Churches are part of traditional African religions because of their character in breaking from Western Christianity and Western colonialism. This transition was observed without deeply reflecting on the possibility of breaking out of colonialism but remaining faithful to the Christian faith. Cabrita (2018:5) explains further that scholars were quick to label ritual healing as non-orthodox without taking into cognizance that this was a way of transforming protestant Christianity but not necessarily breaking from the Christian faith. Therefore, moving away from mainline Christianity was interpreted as alignment to traditional African religions without the fact that there has been schism in Christianity over the years which did not necessarily signify the misalignment from the Christian faith. Cabrita (2018:5) explains that in the South African context scholars are quick to link ritual healing to traditional healing without the ability to distinguish between the two. Consequently, a prophet in African Independent Churches would be seen in the same way as a diviner in traditional African religions. The critics of African Independent

Churches got it wrong on this since it is the difference between the diviner and the prophet that gave rise to healing in African Independent Churches whereby these churches did not only win people coming from mainline Christianity but also from traditional African religions.

The main argument in this book is that ritual healing in African Independent Churches such as Zion Christian Church needs to be distinguished from traditional African medicine. While both types of healing may rely on symbols, ceremonies and rituals, they differ significantly in their source and spirituality. The ritual healing process in the Zion Christian Church is linked to the Christian faith, while traditional African medicine is linked to traditional African religious practices. This is how Bishop Barnabas Lekganyane during his keynote address at the Humboldt-University of Berlin quoted by Stork and Du Toit (2022:203) explained the differences when he said:

> I have observed with disappointment misconceptions of the tolerance of cultures and customs that the ZCC practices, being confused with promoting ancestral worship and other customary practices forbidden in the Bible. As a church, we respect people's identities, cultures, and customs. However, we do not practice or encourage the practicing of aspects of traditions related to ancestral worship and healing through traditional medicines. While those who themselves believe in traditional healing and ancestral worship are welcome to attend our church services, as is everyone else, members of the church are not allowed to participate in ceremonies of ancestral worship, traditional initiation schools, and to use traditional medicines.

Cabrita (2018:130) concurs with the bishop because 'affiliating with Zion meant decisively breaking with the older order of health and healing represented by traditional healers, chiefs, and local patriarchs. Embracing divine healing meant cutting oneself off from one's ancestors. No longer could a Zion convert make sacrifices to their ancestral spirits.' These distinctions will be discussed in detail in the chapters to follow in the book by demonstrating how the various healing rituals in the Zion Christian Church such as healing, protection, worship, prophecy and taboos differ from the practices in traditional African medicine.

An autoethnographic study on the ritual healing process

This book is an autoethnographic study of the ritual healing process in the Zion Christian Church. Adams, Ellis and Jones (2017:1) define an autoethnography as a 'form of ethnographic research in which a researcher connects personal experiences to wider cultural, political, and social meanings and understandings'. In this book, autoethnography is relevant because I have as the author been deeply immersed in the ritual healing process of the Zion Christian Church over many years. I have also immersed myself in the practices of the church, its customs, traditions, spirituality and culture in the African context. I was born in the Zion Christian Church and grew up in the church until I was fourteen years old. These experiences will form part of my analysis of the ritual healing process in the Zion Christian Church. Other than my experiences and encounters with the Zion Christian Church, the available literature (secondary data) on the ritual healing process in the Zion Christian Church will also serve as part of the analysis of the data collected for this book.

Data will be analysed by using thematic analysis to understand the different themes, prophecy, worship, spiritual protection and social restrictions about the process of ritual healing. For example, on the theme of prophecy, it will be possible to evaluate and understand its different practices. Braun and Clarke (2006:77) state, 'Thematic analysis is a qualitative research method that involves identifying, analysing, and interpreting patterns of meaning (or "themes") within qualitative data.' In this book, the thematic analysis is used in the first place to identify the patterns of the ritual healing process in the Zion Christian Church. In the second instance, this analysis method is used to interpret these patterns concerning the disconnections between traditional African medicine and the ritual healing process in the Zion Christian Church in South Africa. This will help in reaching a broader understanding of the ritual healing process in the African Independent Churches.

An overview of the book

Chapter 2 introduces the foundation of the Zion Christian Church, looking back to the inception of the organization. The available accounts vary concerning when the church started, so this chapter will look at the various possibilities and offer possible dates for the foundation of the Zion Christian Church. The chapter will also look at the founders of the church and its leadership over the years. The chapter further examines the links between this church and the early Pentecostal movement in South Africa. This will be expounded by looking, in the first instance, at Edward Motaung's Pentecostal roots and, in the second instance, at the connection between the Zion Christian Church and the Zion Apostolic Faith Mission. To understand the theological discourses of this church concerning ritual healing, there is a need to look at the links between the Zion Christian Church and the Zionism of John Alexander Dowie. The Zion Christian Church is discussed here as one of the African Independent Churches. The church will also be discussed as part of the broader African Zionism Movement, which has strong foundations in Zionism. Lastly, the chapter will look at the broader membership in the Zion Christian Church and the various branches that exist throughout the world to understand this church as one of the largest African Independent Churches. These historical developments of the church are important in the understanding of the ritual healing process in the Zion Christian Church.

Chapter 3 identifies a variety of purification rituals in the Zion Christian Church by using the ritual healing theory to trace the origin of healing in this church. One of the purification rituals in the Zion Christian Church is the use of prayer by the church leader or pastor. The minister will use a piece of wood (*kotana*) and a sheet of paper to be waved rapidly over the patient's body. Secondly, the church uses blessed coffee and blessed tea in the healing of individuals. Thirdly, holy water is also used after it has been prayed over by the pastor or the church leader. The fourth healing practice in the Zion Christian Church is the pricking of the skin using a needle that has been prayed over by the minister in the church and that can be applied to the nose, the hands and the legs. The last healing practice is the use of salted water for the cleansing of the body and purification. This is applied to induce either vomiting or diarrhea. Therefore, the members of the Zion Christian Church are used to what they call *o berekisha mala* for diarrhea or *o kapa* for vomiting. Both practices are used to maintain purification in the body of the believer by taking away any unwanted substances. All five of these practices are discussed here to bring an understanding of the disconnections between traditional African medicine and ritual healing in the Zion Christian Church.

Chapter 4 looks at the various symbols and practices of protection in the Zion Christian Church. These are used as it is believed that they can bring protection to the members of the church and also prevent illnesses and diseases. The first protective practice is the sprinkling of water around the home of the believer. This should be differentiated from the water used for healing or even the salted water used to induce diarrhea or vomiting. Secondly, the church badge, which is given to an individual immediately after the water baptism, is also used to protect members of the church in addition to serving as a sign of their faithfulness to and affiliation with the church. Thirdly, the ropes and strings or strips of cloth worn around the body are also believed to have protective powers. Strips of blue cloth, known as *khutane*, have to be worn in a secret place to protect believers against assaults and lightning. Fourthly, the members of the Zion Christian Church also use brown paper to protect themselves against non-members, particularly during visitations. Lastly, the chapter discusses the copper wires that the Zion Christian Church put around the gates of their houses as a means of protecting them from witchcraft. These practices are discussed to highlight the distinctions between traditional African medicine and protective systems in the Zion Christian Church.

Chapter 5 is an exploration of the therapeutic worship in the Zion Christian Church. Worship (including songs and music) using ritual healing theory can become therapeutic. This aspect of the Zion Christian Church is discussed here to show that the singing of hymns and other songs brings healing to the congregants. Praise and worship form an integral part of the liturgy in the Zion Christian Church and form part of the various ceremonies in the church. The different forms of worship are discussed here, together with these ceremonies, to bring disconnections between traditional African medicine and ritual healing. Firstly, the chapter discusses the male choir (also known as *mokhukhu*) whose worship practices have healing implications. Secondly, the chapter explores the practices of the female choir, the worship practices of which also have similar healing implications. Thirdly, both the male and female choirs are active in the *mpoho* ceremony, which involves dancing and singing throughout the night. Fourthly, the Zion Christian Church believes in different kinds of gatherings that are also used to offer prayers for the sick to receive healing in their lives. Lastly, the sermon which is offered in the branches of the church during Sunday services in particular brings healing to their lives. Moreover, it is the sermon ministered by preachers in this church that is also expected to bring healing to the people of God in this church. These matters are discussed here as part of the therapeutic practices within the context of praise and worship in the church.

Chapter 6 studies the matter of therapeutic prophecy and instructions in the Zion Christian Church. The prophecy in the Zion Christian Church is given to individuals by calling them out and addressing them privately rather than in public. The Zion Christian Church uses a diagnostic prophecy whereby the prophet reveals the various causative factors to the sicknesses and diseases happening in the life of the believer. However, prophecy is not only the diagnosis but also a prediction of the future with events that are supposed to happen in the future being foretold in the present. This chapter will also look at some of the prophecies that are given in this church aimed at addressing the problems of witchcraft and misfortunes. The chapter will explain the role of the Holy Spirit in the diagnosis of the problem during prophecy in the Zion Christian Church. After being able to diagnose the problem with the help of the Holy Spirit, the prophet will then give prophetic instructions for dealing with the problem. These various practices of prophecy are identified and discussed here as part of the examination of the healing implications of prophecy in the Zion Christian Church. The chapter argues that prophecy in the Zion Christian Church should be differentiated from divination in traditional African religions.

Chapter 7 looks at the social restrictions and taboos in the Zion Christian Church, which have therapeutic and protective implications for the life of the believer. The Zion Christian Church has many taboos which, in a way, contribute to the well-being of its believers. Among the taboos or restrictions in the Zion Christian Church are those on food, particularly the prohibition on eating pork or the meat of animals that died of natural illness. The women in this church are expected to dress respectfully for their well-being. The chapter will also discuss the fact that smoking and drinking are discouraged, particularly among the church's ministers. Other restrictions exist in the church about death, as well as how funerals should be conducted and how members should behave during such ceremonies. There are also restrictions on the unveiling of tombstones of the members of the church. Members of the church whose children have attended initiation schools are not supposed to go to church for a certain number of weeks. The Zion Christian Church itself is considered a sacred place with many restrictions, particularly regarding visitors who must obtain prior permission before visiting their premises. The practices of these social restrictions and taboos are too different from practices in the traditional African religions.

The last chapter is a summary of findings on the ritual healing process in the Zion Christian Church. This chapter revisits all the aspects of the ritual healing process in the church such as healing rituals, protective rituals, worship rituals, prophecy rituals, social restrictions and taboos to differentiate them from traditional African medicine. This chapter warns against the demonization and paganization of the ritual healing process in the Zion Christian Church and other African Independent Churches. Theologians and scholars of religious studies, anthropology, history and other disciplines should be able to make distinctions between traditional African medicine and the use of healing rituals to avoid generalization and condemnation of the African Independent churches for using the latter.

2

Zion Christian Church: An overview

Introduction

This chapter introduces the foundation of the Zion Christian Church since its inception. It is uncertain when the church started, and this chapter will look at the various possibilities and offer possible foundation dates of the Zion Christian Church. The chapter will also look at the founders of the church, its leadership over the years, and the links between this church and the early Pentecostal movement in South Africa. This will be expounded by investigating Church leaders' Pentecostal roots and the connection between the Zion Christian Church and the fundamental teachings of Pentecostalism. To understand the theological discourses of the church concerning healing and taboos, links between the Zion Christian Church and the Zionism of John Alexander Dowie should be studied. The Zion Christian Church is discussed here as an African Independent Church; hence, various characteristics of African Independent Churches are highlighted. The church will also be discussed as part of the broader African Zionism movement with strong foundations in Zionism. Lastly, the chapter will explore the growth of the Zion Christian Church and the various branches that exist throughout the world to understand that this church is one of the largest African Independent Churches. The rationale behind the growth of the Zion Christian Church will be explained in this regard. The historical developments of the church are important in the understanding of the ritual healing process in the Zion Christian Church. It also helps to grasp the broader sense of the ritual healing process in the African Independent Churches. In addition, it demonstrates the Christian roots of the church as opposed to the roots of traditional African religions.

Early developments of the Zion Christian Church

There are two Zion Christian Churches in South Africa, the Star and Saint Engenas (the Dove). In this study, the focus is on the Star, which is situated in Moria, Polokwane, Limpopo province. The Zion Christian Church is the largest African Independent Church in South Africa and the second largest church on the continent (Brockman 2011:341; Bongmba 2015:555; Sanneh & McClymond 2016). The Church was founded by Ignatius (popularly known as Engenas) Lekganyane. Engenas was born in 1885 in a village called Thabakgone near Mamabolo in Northern Transvaal (now Limpopo province), South Africa, and died in 1948 (Clarke 2004, Morton 2018). In 1910 Engenas received a vision to start the church in which he saw many people following him. Many leaders in the African Independent Churches receive their calling through visions and dreams. Although the year 1910 is widely accepted by some leaders and followers of the Church as the starting date of the Zion Christian Church, Elias Khebeleni Lukhaimane (1980) in his Master's dissertation completed at the University of the North argues that the church did not immediately start in 1910. The main reason is that between 1910 and 1924, the founding father of the Zion Christian Church, Engenas was involved in various activities outside Thabakgone; therefore, it is very unlikely that he would have started the Church at that time. One such activity, according to Lukhaimane (1980:6), is that Engenas had another vision in 1912 where he was told to leave Thabakgone, Mamabolo to go to Johannesburg where he was supposed to join a church that baptizes people in a three-times immersion. On arrival in Johannesburg, Engenas met the Mahlangu brothers, Elias and Joseph, who one day when they were baptizing people followed the three-times immersion as in Engenas' dream. Engenas was then baptized by the Mahlangu brothers and was part of the Zion Apostolic Church (ZAC) in Johannesburg until 1917. It is also widely accepted that in the five years, between 1912 and 1917, while in Johannesburg, Engenas met many great leaders in the Zionist movement including Pieter le Roux and other Black Zionist leaders.

In 1918 Engenas became the ordained leader of the branch of Mahlangu's Zion Apostolic Church in his village in Thabakgone, Mamabolo. Since his ordination, he could baptize people using the same method of triple immersion. During this year Engenas won many converts because he was a powerful preacher. Engenas also had great prophetic gifts. He could predict the future, and this included Germany's defeat by Britain which happened in 1917. Lukhaimane (1980:10) explains that Engenas got married in 1918 and continued to work with the Mahlangu brothers. Elias Mahlangu was the Superintendent of the Zion Apostolic Church with its headquarters in Johannesburg. However, according to Lukhaimane (1980:10), Engenas was not happy with some of the practices of the Zion Apostolic Church such as wearing long white robes, for men to grow their beards, and for adherents to take off their shoes when entering the premises of the church. Other than the doctrinal differences between Engenas and the Mahlangus, there were also challenges of power between these leaders because Engenas was excelling in his gift of prophecy. Engenas could predict the events of the future and had a great following because of his charisma. Lukhaimane (1980:11) thinks that the Mahlangu brothers thought that they would be overshadowed by Engenas' great gifts to a level of insignificance. These differences caused Engenas to finally break away from the Zion Apostolic Church in 1920.

In the same year, following the breakaway from the Mahlangus, Engenas joined Edward Motaung's Zion Apostolic Faith Mission whose headquarters was in Lesotho (Lukhaimane 1980:32). Motaung who is also known as 'the lion' was a powerful preacher with great gifts of healing and performing miracles. It seems to me that Engenas admired the greatness of Motaung as he was also a highly gifted preacher. Engenas was then ordained as the Bishop of the Zion Apostolic Faith Mission for the work in the Northern Transvaal (Lukhaimane 1980:12). The Zion Apostolic Faith Mission was also a Pentecostal church that had split with the main Apostolic Faith Mission. But soon after joining Motaung, challenges started to emerge between the two leaders. The differences between Lekganyane and Motaung were not necessarily doctrinal as was the case with the Mahlangus Zion Apostolic Church. Anderson (1999:289) points out that 'Lekganyane's marriage to a second wife was one reason for the break with Motaung, who opposed polygyny'. Other reasons as pointed out by Lukhaimane (1980:14) related to the issues of positions and a power struggle between Engenas and Motaung. Lukhaimane (1980:14) explains that the Zion Apostolic Faith Mission in the Northern Transvaal was doing well including financially, and this did not sit well with Motaung who summoned Engenas to Lesotho about other administrative issues. This was the last time that Engenas visited Lesotho as he was dissatisfied with the way Motaung handled the matter. It seems to me that Engenas was always longing for autonomy and founding his church; hence, he always struggled to submit to the leadership of leaders such as the Mahlangu brothers and Edward Motaung. It might also be because God had already told him through a vision in 1910 that he would start his church, and hence, he was not fulfilled under the supervision of the Mahlangus and Motaung. Thus, the quest for sole authority continued from 1917 until 1924 when Engenas finally broke his association with Edward Motaung.

At the end of 1924 or the beginning of 1925, according to Anderson (1999:289), Lekganyane started his church, the 'Zion Christian Church' in Thabakgone, Moria, Northern Transvaal (which is now called Limpopo province). The Church in the Northern Transvaal grew and had a great following because some of the adherents of the Zion Apostolic Church and the Zion Apostolic Faith Mission followed him when he started the Zion Christian Church. Another reason for the growth in the early days was the great gifts of prophecy and healing that Engenas used to attract a great following. Anderson (1999:289) points out that when Engenas made the first application to register the church, it had about 1000 adherents. The application to register the Church was not successful at this time given that the government was suspicious of the independent churches which practised racial segregation at that time. In 1930, according to Lukhaimane (1980:21), Engenas also faced another challenge. This time it came from his former leaders at the Zion Apostolic Church who argued that he could no longer use a building that he built while serving under them. Engenas argued that he built the church using his own money and was therefore entitled to continue using it. The matter was discussed in the local tribal council where Engenas was told to leave the Thabakgone, Mamabolo area. According to Anderson (1999:288): 'With the help of attorneys [Lekganyane] was able to buy a farm in Boyne, fifty kilometers east of Pietersburg [now Polokwane]. Church members raised the purchase price and gave the farm to Lekganyane as his personal property.' It was here that the Church's headquarters, formally known as Moria, was built. The city of Zion as it is now called is similar to John Alexander Dowie's Zion city in Chicago. It was later recognized as a sacred place. Adherents of the Church would undertake pilgrimages to the city of Zion to worship God. The idea of Zion City is an eschatological city where there will be no sickness and disease. People will live in peace and harmony, and the sick will be healed.

The Church continued to grow since its inception in 1924, and in ten years, it was a force that could not be ignored in the context of the African Independent Churches. Ten years later, around 1935, the membership of the Zion Christian Church was more than 50,000. It had more than fifty congregations across Southern Africa which made it the biggest church in the region if not the continent (Anderson 1999:290). It is an amazing achievement for a church to grow that much in ten years. This speaks to the great calling and gifts of its leader, Engenas Lekganyane. In addition, the idea of having the headquarters in Boyne and Engenas serving as the main leader who is more of a liberator and prophetic figure contributed towards this growth. This is because power and authority were centralized in one place. It must be reiterated that Engenas had great gifts and power to heal the sick, and he was reluctant to delegate this power to the next generation of leaders or the branch leaders of his church. He wished to keep the power and authority to himself and based at the headquarters. Healing and the performance of miracles took place during the ministry of Engenas Lekganyane. Anderson (1999:290) points out the healing of cripples, barrenness, provision of employment, rainmaking and other miracles as some of the acts that attracted many people to the Zion Christian Church. Because of the performance of these miracles, prophecies and other healing practices, Engenas became very popular in Africa and elsewhere in the world. Engenas Lekganyane died in 1948 after a long illness.

The leadership in the Zion Christian Church

After Engenas Lekganyane's death, it was not clear who should become the main leader of the Zion Christian Church. The constitution (1946) article (iii) elections which was drafted two years before the death of Engenas Lekganyane is not clear on the succession plan except to indicate that the bishop will be elected during an annual conference:

> The Conference shall then proceed to elect a Bishop who shall hold office for life.
>
> The Bishop so elected shall preside at the Annual Conference; shall be recognised as Head of the Church, its executive officer, and the legal representative of the Conference and shall act in all matters on behalf of the church and shall be chairman of all Committees of the Church.

What also made matters worse about the succession plan is that while ideally, the firstborn would be an appropriate successor, the challenge in this instance is that Engenas's firstborn, Barnabas Lekganyane, had died (Moripe 1996:24). Engenas Lekganyane had two sons, Edward Lekganyane (second son) and Joseph Lekganyane (fifth born). This led to a schism where Joseph Lekganyane became the leader of the Zion Christian Church (the Dove). This book does not go into depth to discuss the schism. However, it is important to point out that in the Zion Christian Church (the Star), Engenas Lekganyane was succeeded by Edward Lekganyane in 1948 who worked in Johannesburg when his father died. Edward was reluctant to take up the leadership position, particularly as the Bishop of the church. According to Lukhaimane (1980:87), his full name was Talane Reuben Lekganyane, but he was popularly known as Edward, a name that his father gave him after Edward Motaung. Edward was born at Thabakgone in 1926. This means that he was only twenty-two years of age when he took over the leadership of the Zion Christian Church. The Church continued to grow under Edward's leadership to the extent that in 1954 the Church had about 80,000 members (Moripe 1996:106). Edward, according to Anderson (1999:291), enrolled for theological training at the Dutch Reformed Church's Stofberg Theological College, and it seems he wanted to restore the Church to its biblical foundation. It was also during Edward's leadership that the idea of a prophetic figure and messiahship became unpopular unlike during the reign of his father. However, this caused Edward to face some criticism, particularly for his association with the Dutch Reformed Church where some began to think that this would lead to the Church losing its connection with the Holy Spirit. Edward's leadership also saw the connection between the Zion Christian Church and the apartheid government which came into power in 1948. This, according to Anderson (1999:292), is because the government saw the African Independent Churches as organizations that enabled the continuation of the apartheid theology which saw the separation of people according to their race. Since the African Independent Churches ministered specifically to the Black people, they were never seen as threats by the apartheid government but rather as enablers of apartheid. Hence, Edward invited the government to Easter celebrations where he would address the government and church and state relations. Edward died in 1967 after a short illness.

After Edward Lekganyane's death, the church's natural successor was his son, Ramarumo Barnabas Lekganyane. He was born in 1954 and was very young at the time of his father's death. At the age of thirteen, although the Church Council confirmed Barnabas as the presiding Bishop, he could not immediately take up the leadership position (Moripe 1996:26). Hence, the church appointed a Superintendent, only known to us as Mr Mohale to lead the church on behalf of the Lekganyane family. However, according to Anderson (1999:293), Mr Mohale was power-hungry, and he was replaced by Mr Letsoalo until Barnabas Lekganyane was mature enough to lead the church. In 1975, on his twenty-first birthday, Barnabas started his responsibilities as the leader of the Zion Christian Church. He is still its leader to date. Barnabas' leadership continued with the same strategy of inviting the apartheid regime leaders including the minister of Bantu affairs, Minister Piet Koornhof to the church. According to Ter Haar (2009:68), the state president at that time, PW Botha also visited the church during the Easter celebrations in 1985. It was during this time that he committed to keeping his father's legacy according to Moripe (1996:26):

> I as the leader of the Zion Christian Church feel proud to announce that, my father, the late Bishop E E Lekganyane, and my grandfather, the late Bishop E B Lekganyane had faith in God. This is proved by the good works they did by founding and building Zion Christian Church up to this strength. Through faith, I will also follow in their footsteps for the good of the church.

However, unlike Edward's leadership, Barnabas denounced the system of apartheid. Anderson (2001:104) points out that the church magazine, *Messenger* quoted Barnabas' sermon where he said, 'The Zion Christian Church and I, as a leader, detest apartheid together with all its discriminatory laws. We also abhor killings and allowing people to starve, especially black people.' This is proof that Barnabas was against the apartheid regime which is different from his father's leadership style. The Zion Christian Church continued to speak against the apartheid regime before the elections in 1994 where leaders such as Mangosutu Buthelezi, FW de Klerk and Nelson Mandela were invited to the celebrations at the church's headquarters (Müller 2016). These leaders could not ignore the Zion Christian Church as the largest African Independent Church. Therefore, the Zion Christian Church can be defined as one of the churches that played a constructive role leading up to the negotiations for a democratic South Africa. The church also played a role in the peace rhetoric during racial divisions in South Africa, given its theology of peace and healing which is one of the fundamental teachings of the church.

The difference between Edward and Barnabas is also seen in the return of this messiahship. During the reign of Barnabas, the notion of the leader as the messiah was resuscitated and he was perceived as the messiah in the same way as the first-generation leader, Engenas Lekganyane. According to Lukhaimane (1980:17), Engenas Lekganyane was perceived as a messiah 'to his underprivileged followers who had come to deliver them from bondage, especially from the horror of superstition and the power wielded by the medicine man'. The followers of this church perceive the leaders of the Zion Christian Church as playing a mediator role more than a pastoral role. This kind of role is also seen in how the Zion Christian Church members pray; they pray to the God of Lekganyane. Although the prayer will always end with God the Father, God the Son and God the Holy Spirit, most members would still quote the God of Lekganyane in their prayers. I also remember that my late father (a Zion Christian Church pastor) would in many of his prayers quote the God of Lekganyane in articulating God's ability to perform signs and wonders. Many other pastors would declare their God as the God of Lekganyane. In addition, some of the songs sung in the Zion Christian Church would praise their leaders, Engenas, Edward and Barnabas. However, according to Anderson (1999:296), the church leaders themselves refuse the notion of being the messiahs. They perceived themselves as the earthly leaders of the church who have been ordained by God to serve the people of God here on earth. We should therefore be able to separate the idolization by followers and some members from how the leaders perceived themselves. Anderson (1999:296) continues to say that praying to the 'God of Lekganyane' should not necessarily be perceived as worship of these leaders but 'simply to place God in the Zion Christian Church context as the God of the African leaders who are with them as he was with the far more remote Abraham, Isaac and Jacob'. Therefore, it can be concluded that the members of the Zion Christian Church do not pray to their leaders but rather acknowledge their leaders as spiritual leaders sent by God to deliver them. The honour given to the leaders should be interpreted as the same honour given to biblical figures such as Abraham, Isaac and Jacob. This separates Zion Christian Church from traditional African medicine in the worship of ancestors.

The leadership of the Lekganyane leaders is also strongly rooted in the performance of miracles, signs and wonders. It is a leadership that is understood in the context of deliverance; thus, all the leaders of the Zion Christian Church are perceived as healers and liberators like Moses. It is the same reason that the Zion Christian Church continued to grow even during the apartheid regime as the Church leaders were seen as the liberators from the oppression the Black people faced. Moreover, the three generations of leaders of the Zion Christian Church should be seen as the ones who confront evil forces in the spiritual realm. This role is different from the one of the traditional healers in traditional African medicine. Nonetheless, these leaders are perceived as having the power to bring healing to those who are oppressed by all kinds of sickness and disease. Even the headquarters of the Church is perceived as a place of healing for those who are sick. In this way, anyone who is sick is supposed to receive healing upon touching the grounds of Boyne, Moria. Anderson (1999:297) explains that Boyne is more like an African Zion 'a place of blessing, of deliverance, of healing in short, the place where divine immanence is keenly felt. It is also the place where the means of grace and the manifestation of God's presence in the sacraments are administered by the bishop.' When sick people arrive in Boyne, they believe that they will receive their healing and deliverance as it is considered a place of grace, healing and deliverance. The conferences at the Zion

Christian Church headquarters are important to the followers as they will allow them such an encounter. Therefore, even the adherents who recently joined the Church also look forward to visiting Boyne immediately after a conference. According to Anderson (1999:297), the Zion Christian Church follows the Old Testament approach when it comes to the celebration of annual festivals. They believe that the followers of the church would have a divine encounter with their God. Therefore, the celebrations of the Zion Christian Church during Easter and in September have the same purpose where believers come to have an encounter with their God.

Zion Christian Church as an African Independent Church

The African Independent Churches' large following is an important contributor to the religious space. Together with the Pentecostal churches in Africa, they have contributed to the shift of the religious influence from the global north to the global south, particularly in Africa. The Zion Christian Church is considered an African Independent Church because it was started independently by an African leader, Engenas Lekganyane, and continued to function without the supervision of Western missionaries. Thus, Lekganyane can also be categorized as a decolonial leader who founded a decolonial church. The word 'Independent' in this context means that no foreign sources have any financial or doctrinal control over them. It also speaks to the autonomy of churches such as the Zion Christian Church in the day-to-day running of the church, including the doctrinal practices. Churches such as the Zion Christian Church started to break away from Western missionary oppression as a resistance to colonial and imperialist oppression which occurred in most churches started by missionaries coming from the global north. Many of the African leaders who served faithfully in the Western missionary churches felt that they had to minister the gospel in a way that would be relevant to the African context. Consequently, many broke away to start the African Independent Churches. The Zion Christian Church should be perceived in the same way as leaders such as Engenas Lekganyane who served in churches such as the Apostolic Faith Mission but later left to minister relevantly to their people. In Western missionary churches, leaders such as Engenas Lekganyane could not be recognized as pastors during the time of racial oppression and colonialism of a special kind in South Africa called apartheid. As a result, they could not function fully with their gifts, but when they started their churches, they were able to minister the gospel and function as prophets.

Therefore, the African Independent Churches are important in presenting the gospel in the African context in a way that Africans can understand the message. The Zion Christian Church started for similar reasons by wanting to appeal to Africans through the ministration of the gospel.

The African Independent Churches such as the Zion Christian Church are defined by a leading scholar in the field, Philomena Mwaura (2004, 2007, 2014) as an African response to Christianity. Churches such as these have challenged us to start looking at Christianity and the presentation of the gospel in light of the religious needs of the African people. Therefore, the Zion Christian Church as an African Independent Church can be considered as the church that has been able to decolonize and Africanize Christian practices by making them relevant to the African context. In these churches, Christianity adapted to the African contexts and began to address the challenges faced by Africans. In addition, they can also be seen as the indigenization of the Christian faith by making it relevant to the African people. Churches like these have given Christianity an African flavour where the Christian tradition is understood and practised in an African context taking into consideration African culture, African customs and African identity. Scholars such as Olupona (2014) describe the Zion Christian Church and other African Independent Churches as churches that have found the balance between the Christian faith and the African culture but not necessarily African Traditional religions. This is why churches like these are popular in the African continent. This is also the reason why people moved from the Western missionary churches to the African Independent Churches such as the Zion Christian Church as they saw signs of decolonization in these churches. Therefore, our understanding of the ritual healing process in the Zion Christian Church begins when we understand this church in light of its Africanness and indigenization. This will assist in understanding the rationale behind some of the healing practices in the Zion Christian Church and other African Independent Churches. And why they do not follow the American-euro centric paradigms in the healing practices but an African approach.

As discussed in Chapter 1 of this book, there are different types of African Independent Churches such as Ethiopian, Zionist, Spirit-type, Aladura and so forth. Anderson (1991:2) explains that there could be many other Zionist-type churches in Africa or the African Independent Church. However, the author shies away from the 'Zionist' category given other reasons or other associations that Zionism has elsewhere in the world. Ordinarily, the Zion Christian Church would also be classified as a Zionist-type African Independent Church, given its name or some Zionist elements. However, leading scholars in the field such as Daneel (1987, 2000, 2001) and Anderson (1999, 2000, 2001, 2018) classify the Zion Christian Church as the Spirit-type African Independent Church because of its alignment with the work of the Holy Spirit in addition to their Zionist practices. I regard the observations of these leading scholars as correct. I have noticed that the members of the Zion Christian Church in the local congregation do also refer to the 'Holy Spirit'. The same happens when a prophet in the local congregation is about to give a prophetic word. The perception is that such a person has been captured by the Holy Spirit, which allows them to utter the revelation of prophecy. Therefore, the African Independent Churches are different from traditional African religions in the belief of the Holy Spirit.

This brings us to the next characteristic of the Spirit-type churches such as the Zion Christian Church, which is the respect for the prophetic figure who is leading the church (Anderson 1991). In the case of the Zion Christian Church, three Bishops in the person of Engenas Lekganyane, Edward Lekganyane and Barnabas Lekganyane are recognized as prophetic figures who possess the gifts of healing and prophecy. These gifts manifested more in the life of Engenas Lekganyane than in the life of Edward and his son Barnabas. As discussed previously, during the reign of Edward, the people accused him of having departed from the pneumatic experiences, particularly when he underwent theological training at the Dutch Reformed Church. During the reign of Barnabas, the church adopted the prophethood of believers and we see ministers in local branches ministering to their local congregants. I have also observed lately that ministers are appointed who can minister prophecies to the local congregants. The size of the church makes it impossible for leaders such as Barnabas Lekganyane to occupy this prophetic role to pray for everyone. The prophetic figure is perceived as the anointed leader who is supposed to lead the ritual healing process or empower other leaders who will do so in local branches of the church. The Lekganyanes are not the only ones who had the gift of healing and prophecy. Similar churches such as Frederick Samuel Modise's International Pentecost Holiness Church (IPHC) and Isaiah Mloyiswa Mdliwamafa Shembe of the Ibandla lamaNazaretha are also recognized as the prophetic figures of their churches with gifts of healing and prophecy. The respect that the followers and members of the African Independent Churches give to their leaders should be understood in the broader perspective of African customs and cultures where a spiritual figure is given respect. This should be differentiated from the worship of ancestors in traditional African religions. Respect for the spiritual leader does not immediately lead to the idolization of the same leader.

African Independent Churches, such as the Zion Christian Church, have given the ritual healing process in the practice of faith healing much attention. African Independent Churches have incorporated other methods of healing such as the use of symbols and objects in healing. Therefore, the Zion Christian Church is considered an African Independent Church because like all other like-minded churches, they use symbols, ceremonies and objects in healing. As discussed in the preceding sections, it is the ministry of healing that has contributed to the rise of the Church in the first quarter of the twentieth century where leaders such as Engenas Lekganyane rose to fame because of their healing ministry. Thus, the healing ministry, particularly the Ritual healing process, is at the centre of the theology of African Independent Churches. These churches are situated mainly in rural areas where many people depend on faith healing compared to, for example, modern medicine. In a way, the African Independent Churches are filling a gap in the context of health where those who cannot afford modern medicine have the option of ritual healing. Thus, the Zion Christian Church is one such African Independent Church that fills that gap in the practice of healing and prophecy. This practice in the church and other African Independent Churches has an indigenous provenance as opposed to conventional methods such as the laying on of hands. The interest in this book lies in the disconnections between traditional African medicine and the ritual healing process in the Zion Christian Church. And how this will help in the development of a theology of ritual healing process in African Independent Churches. I will demonstrate in the following chapters that the use of healing rituals does not always lead to traditional African medicine as ritual healing is not originally religious but simply depends on how the religious group uses it. Thus, African Independent Churches, I would argue, use the healing rituals within the precinct of the Christian faith, while traditional African medicine uses the same healing rituals as part of the traditional African religious practices. In the next section, I look at the intersections between the Zion Christian Church and Pentecostalism.

Zion Christian Church and Pentecostalism

There are links between the Zion Christian Church and the early development of the Pentecostal movement in South Africa. As discussed above, the link between the Zion Christian Church and Pentecostalism is seen in the encounters between the founder of the church, Engenas Lekganyane, and one of the leaders of the Apostolic Faith Mission, Pieter le Roux. In the first instance, Engenas arrived in Johannesburg around 1908 to seek healing because of his eye disorder (Anderson 1999:287). It was owing to his search for healing that he had an encounter with Pentecostalism. It is important to point out that at this time the founder of the Apostolic Faith Mission, John G. Lake, arrived in South Africa, and it is highly probable that Engenas had met with the founding father of Pentecostalism. In the second instance, during his stay in Johannesburg in the years between 1912 and 1917, he came into contact with the Apostolic Faith Mission through Pieter le Roux who led the church after John G. Lake returned to the United States of America. In the third instance, Engenas experienced Pentecostalism through the Mahlangu brothers, Elias and Joseph, before they started the Zion Apostolic Church (Anderson 1999:287). Therefore, it is correct to point out that Engenas, the founding Bishop of Zion Christian Church, was part of the largest classical Pentecostal church, the Apostolic Faith Mission in its early development. It is also correct to point out that in the early stages of the Zion Christian Church, Engenas followed the fundamental teachings of the Pentecostal movement including baptism in the Holy Spirit and the gift of speaking in tongues. It was during this period that he learned of baptism through triple immersion. These historical developments place the founder and the church itself as a movement that is deeply rooted in the Christian tradition, particularly Pentecostalism. In addition, these further demonstrate the association with Christianity and dissociation with traditional African religions.

The church began the ministry of healing through the ordinary method of the laying on of hands like many other Pentecostals. However, as the church grew it became impossible to lay hands on everyone (Anderson 1999:290). It seems that Engenas began the use of the blessed water to reach out to as many sick people as he could. Engenas did not adopt this method in joining the traditional African religions but in a quest to reach as many people as he could. The leaders after Engenas, namely Edward and Barnabas then began to emulate their predecessors by using anointed objects in the Ritual healing process but again not as a deviation from Christian practices but to reach many of their followers and members. Therefore, the issue of how to pray for the many adherents of the Zion Christian Church led to the doctrinal differences between classical Pentecostal churches and the church. From the second generation of leaders such as Edward Lekganyane, it became normal practice in the church to bless water and other material things for healing purposes. But it also speaks to the idea that Engenas wanted to retain the indigenous provenance in faith healing in the Zion Christian Church. The congregants believed that God had given all the powers to Engenas;

hence, they began to honour him as the main leader of the church. However, the fact that the practices of healing in the Zion Christian Church differ in approach from those of classical Pentecostal churches does not immediately make them similar to traditional African medicine. As I highlighted before, it is probable to use ritual healing independent of traditional African medicine.

After all, as much as there are differences between classical Pentecostal churches and the Zion Christian Church, there are also some similarities. It is important to point out that both the Zion Christian Church and the classical Pentecostal Churches believe in baptism by triple immersion, which is also baptism in the name of the Father, the Son and the Holy Spirit. This is something that Engenas treasured the most as he saw this in a dream and was able to confirm that God indeed wanted him to baptize people through triple immersion. This aspect strengthened the connections between Pentecostalism and Zionism in South Africa. The Trinitarian formula in water baptism, that is, baptism in the name of the Father, the Son and the Holy Spirit is also scriptural as Christ himself commanded his disciple to conduct baptism similarly (Matthew 28:19). Thus, this is something that the Zion Christian Church has treasured over the years as it not only connected them with Pentecostalism but also aligns with the scriptures. However, the Zion Christian Church normally conducts its baptism in running water, which is not common among classical Pentecostals. The latter would rather conduct their baptismal services in the baptism pool. The Zion Christian Church is not the only church that uses baptism in running water. Other African Independent Churches also baptize in running water, and it is believed that this has significance in healing and deliverance. It is believed among African Independent Churches that running water casts out evil spirits during baptism. Therefore, rather than baptize in baptism pools, the African Independent Churches such as the Zion Christian Church baptize believers in running water with the same belief that they will receive their healing and deliverance during the experience. In addition, baptism in the Zion Christian Church also serves as part of the ritual healing process. It is believed that during the baptism experience, sickness and diseases would depart and be cast into the water. Again we see some parallels between the Zion Christian Church and the classical Pentecostals church which also proves the dissociations with traditional African religions.

There is also a commonality between Zionism and Pentecostalism in the sense that both believe in pneumatic experiences, particularly the gift of prophecy and speaking in tongues. Although the Zion Christian Church does not put much emphasis on the baptism of the Holy Spirit, it nonetheless refers to the Spirit. The Spirit in the Zion Christian Church and the Holy Spirit in classical Pentecostalism empower the prophet to prophesy. Anderson (1999:297) states that 'those participating in the religious activity in the Zion Christian Church directly attribute much of that activity to the working of the Holy Spirit. He is the one who gives revelations to the prophets and causes them to behave 'abnormally' with jerking, jumping, snorting and various other contortions of the body.' It is correct to point out that the gift of prophecy in the Zion Christian Church is interpreted as a pneumatic gift that only comes as the result of having an encounter with the Holy Spirit. The prophet is perceived as someone who has the gift of the Holy Spirit which enables him to receive revelations of things in the spirit realm. The Zion Christian Church does not emphasize speaking in tongues, but few among the believers, particularly those with the gift of prophecy, speak in tongues. It is common among the prophets in the Zion Christian Church to quote the word 'maita, maita' when they prophesy. In my opinion, these pneumatic experiences are informed by the encounters Engenas Lekganyane had in the classical Pentecostal churches such as the Apostolic Faith Mission as the latter was founded on the encounter with God through the baptism of the Holy Spirit and the gift of speaking in tongues. Again this demonstrates the Christian roots of the Zion Christian Church rather than the popular connections that some scholars make between the church and African Traditional religions. However, scholars such as Sundkler (1961), Hanekom (1975) and Mokgobi (2014) have mistakenly confused these pneumatic experiences as similar to those in the traditional African religions.

The influence of John Alexander Dowie

There is a clear connection between the Zionist movement of John Alexander Dowie and the Zion Christian Church in South Africa. John Alexander Dowie was born in 1847 and died in 1907. He was an influential leader when it came to the teachings of Zionism. He was the founder of the Christian Catholic Apostolic Church in 1896, which was situated in what he called 'Zion City' near Chicago. Dowie believed in leadership as being directed by God, and he also believed in an Apostolic type of leadership where he was regarded by his followers as an Apostle. Alexander Dowie believed in faith healing where he would teach his followers not to rely too much on Western medicine. Cabrita (2018:1) explains that 'Zion was a worldwide faith-healing movement that instructed its working-class followers to pray for bodily health and to renounce medical assistance'. Dowie also taught his followers several restrictions and taboos, much of which became part of the ritual observance in the Zion Christian Church in South Africa. He was known as the minister of healing throughout his life until he died in 1907 (Sundkler 1976:30; cf. Kgatle 2016:163). Dowie had a vision to start a branch of his church in South Africa, but because of his commitments in Zion City in Chicago, he could not start this work himself. As a result, Dowie delegated Daniel Bryant to come to South Africa to start the work on his behalf. Bryant like his mentor, Dowie, was also committed to the teachings of the Zionist movement. He and his wife were committed to the work of ministry for many years (Sundkler 1976:34; cf. Kgatle 2016:166). Therefore, the influence of the Zionist movement led by Alexander Dowie related very much to the arrival of Daniel Bryant in South Africa. It is also correct to say that the Zionist movement influenced many other churches in South Africa and the rest of the continent, particularly the early inception of Zionism at the beginning of the twentieth century (Nel 2020:11). Alexander Dowie had a big influence on what is today known as the African Zionism movement. However, the reference to this influence should in no way be interpreted as making churches such as Zion Christian Church branches of Dowie. In other words, even with great influence from leaders such as Dowie, the Zion Christian Church should still be described as an African Independent Church.

In 1904, upon his arrival in South Africa, Daniel Bryant met Pieter le Roux who was part of the Dutch Reformed Church but had seceded with a group of about 150 members. This group became part of the Zionist movement in what is popularly known as the Wakkerstroom Congregation which was situated in what was known as the Eastern Transvaal then. Nel (2005:206) explains that 'Bryant and Le Roux led a procession of hundreds of black Zionist members through the streets of Wakkerstroom. Bryant also baptized 141 persons in the river, including Le Roux and his wife.' Bryant later ordained Pieter le Roux to become the elder of the Christian Catholic Apostolic Church in Zion and his wife the evangelist. Most of the Black Zionist churches' leaders came from this congregation. This church therefore had a big influence on the Zion Christian Church as leaders such as the Mahlangu brothers, and Engenas Lekganyane himself can be linked to this congregation. Similarly, Edward Motaung who, as set out in the preceding sections, influenced Engenas Lekganyane was once a member of this congregation. Other important early Black Zionist leaders of the Zionist movement included Daniel Nkonyane, Paul Mabilitsa and Titus Msibi (Khorommbi 2001:20).

Cabrita (2018:2) tells a 'story of transatlantic Zion, an international evangelical Christian faith-healing church that originated in Australia, and subsequently spread from the United States across the Atlantic Ocean to become what is now the single largest religious movement of modern Southern Africa'. However, some scholars make distinctions between the Zionist movement of John Alexander Dowie in the United States and the Zionist movement in Africa. One such scholar is Etherington (1979:125), who states that the main difference between these two movements is that in Africa Zionism in churches such as the Zionist Christian Church has the indigenous foundations which incorporate the cultural aspects. The point made by Etherington does not necessarily mean that these churches deviate much from the Bible or the theological foundation of their practices but rather point out that they connect the same with their African culture. This connection with the indigenous knowledge system demonstrates more of the indigenization of Christianity which is different from the mixing of religious beliefs, that is, syncretism. Khorommbi (2001:20) concurs: 'Although the beginnings of the African Zionist movement have some links with Dowie's movement and White members, the actual African Zionist groups of churches have always been founded by Africans themselves since then.' As pointed out previously, this means that we should be able to point to the similarities between the Zionist movement by Dowie and the African Zionist movement without giving away the uniqueness and independence of the latter. According to De Wet (1989:35), this also speaks to the fact that the African Zionist churches, such as the Zionist Christian Church, were started by African leaders without any contribution financially or otherwise by foreign movements. This speaks volumes in how the African Zionist movement is comprised of churches that have characteristics of the teachings of Zionism but did not necessarily duplicate the American version. Cabrita (2018:5) concurs that 'Zion in Southern Africa developed uniquely local features including the prominent figure of the prophet from the mid-twentieth-century on, something largely absent from the North American tradition'.

One of the similarities between the Zionist churches in Africa and the American version of Zionism is the focus on healing and prophecy, which was the teachings of John Alexander Dowie as discussed above. Most if not all the Zionist churches in Africa similar to the Zion Christian Church teach about faith healing. In addition, according to Oosthuizen (2000:1101), they are known for 'purification rites and taboos as the main means of expression of their faith'. These purification rites and taboos are also observed in the quest to live a holy life which is one of the prerequisites of obtaining divine health. The observance of purification rites and the observance of taboos are also part of a ritual healing process. Ranger (2007:65) thinks that these differences have assisted the Zionist movement in Africa to have its unique characteristics and maintain an African culture in their religious practices. It is for the same reason that at the beginning of the twentieth century, the Zionist movement in South Africa became a source of religious independence which also differentiated them from the missional churches in the context of Pentecostalism. According to Khathide (2010:46), the Zionist churches in South Africa became the option for many Black people who wanted to express their Christian belief in an African way, which they could not do when they were under the Western missionary churches. This led to the proliferation of the Zionist churches in that period, hence their growth over the years. Therefore, the ability of the Zion Christian Church to express Christianity in an African way demonstrates that it is a true African church. The main argument I make here and in the rest of the book is that these indigenous expressions of the gospel in healing, worship and prophecy should not be associated with the practices of traditional African religions. In the next section, I explain the rationale for the growth of the Zionist churches, particularly the Zion Christian Church in South Africa.

The rationale for the growth of the Zion Christian Church

As discussed in the first section of this chapter, the Zion Christian Church is the largest African Independent church in South Africa and the second largest on the continent. It is a powerful church influencing the religious landscape on the African continent. According to the 2011 census, the church's membership of around 5 million contributes almost 50% of the membership of the African Independent es of 10 million and 10% of the Christian population in South Africa. There is no doubt that the Zion Christian Church is one of the most influential churches in the country and on the continent alike. This church has become a religious centre in Africa, and its conferences have become so popular that people travel from different countries to visit the headquarters of the Zion Christian Church in Moria. The million members of the Zion Christian Church frequent these conferences, particularly during the Easter celebrations. Even though leadership has changed over the years, the church has not stopped growing. It can be said that this church is dominant in rural areas where many people rely on prayer for healing as opposed to modern healing. However, I have observed that there are large numbers of people from the cities who frequent the church in villages and townships in search of prayers. Therefore, it is more correct to say that the Zion Christian Church is influential in both rural and urban areas. In addition, one can point out that both the poor and the rich have found the Zion Christian Church attractive in the context of religious needs. However, for this book, it is important to look at the contributing factors towards the growth and influence of the Zion Christian Church.

One of the contributing factors of the Zion Christian Church is its ability to incorporate African culture and customs in its religious practices (Anderson 2001:107). The Zion Christian Church as well as other African Independent Churches combine the elements of African culture and Christianity in their religious practices. The Zion Christian Church can be considered a blended church with some Christian theology, Pentecostalism and African culture. This might be considered something that has assisted the Church in finding resonance among many Africans. This is one of the strengths of the Zion Christian Church since the majority of Africans do not want to abandon their culture as part of their Christian practices. Thus, the Zion Christian Church becomes a fertile ground through which African culture and customs are part of religious practices. In the end, the church can attract a great following because of this balance. The Zion Christian Church is very much African in its approach to doing church in its spiritual experiences and liturgical practices. Its Africanity has contributed to its growth and is an important factor in the ritual healing process. This religious hybridity of the Zion Christian Church I argue should not be confused with the mixing of different religious beliefs.

The Zion Christian Church is very attractive to the African people when it comes to worship. Songs and music in this church reflect much of African liturgy compared to the Western Christian missionary churches that resemble their foundation in Europe (Anderson 2001:107). Therefore, this church has cut the umbilical cord with the colonial matrix of power even when it comes to worship. In the Zion Christian Church, it is not only about the singing, but there is also an incorporation of African dance styles in their liturgy. The choir's song and dance in the Zion Christian Church are all rooted in the African styles of worship. The songs being sung in the Zion Christian Church are also very popular with non-adherents of the church, and some are attracted by the music. Again, it is important to point out that the many segments of the Zion Christian Church music are connected to the cultural practices that many Africans are already familiar with; hence, they find the music attractive. Rafapa (2013) argues that most of the music in the Zion Christian Church follows popular African music. Hence, it is culturally infected music. In addition, much of the music in the Zion Christian Church is sung under the influence of the Holy Spirit which makes it very touching music and attractive to the listeners. The argument here is that their love for music attracts a large number of members to the church. However, the message of their songs remains biblical and aimed at ministering healing to the followers and the members of the church.

The pneumatic practices of prophecy are also major contributing factors to the growth of the Zion Christian Church and other African Independent Churches. Prophecy in the Zion Christian Church is practised with the combination of the revelations of dreams and visions that members find very attractive (Anderson 2001:107). The message of God is not only transmitted through the presentation of the sermon as done in the Western missionary churches but also through visions and dreams (Anderson 2001:107). Therefore, dreams and visions also become an aspect of spirituality in African independent churches that demonstrate African aspects of these churches. Some of the members of the church would join the church because of revelations they received in their dreams and visions. Given the role of dreams and visions in African cosmology, when someone receives confirmation to join the church through the same, they are convinced that they have indeed made the correct decision. Hence, I have observed that members of the Zion Christian Church have been loyal to the church for many years. It is also important to point out that in the Zion Christian Church, prophecy is more than the delivered word of God through visions and dreams. It is also connected to healing which is also another point of attraction. This is considered by scholars such as Daneel (2019) and Anderson (2001) as one of the main reasons why people join the Zion Christian Church. They seek the prophetic word that not only gives them a direction in life but is also able to bring healing to their lives. A prophet figure is seen as someone who can deliver the word from God and interpret congregants' dreams and visions. Most importantly, and as discussed before, the prophet figure in the Zion Christian Church is someone who is expected to have healing powers. The prophet is also someone who can discern the movement of the Holy Spirit or spirit and can give direction to the rest of the congregants when such happens during the spiritual service. Anderson (2001:108) explains that it is believed that the Holy Spirit manifests in a supernatural way on the prophets to operate in the prophetic where the various challenges that the people go through are revealed to the prophets. In addition, the prophet would be able to give certain instructions to help the patient under the same influence of the Holy Spirit. Here we see the links between diagnostic prophecy and healing. This too is a valid reason for the people in Africa to join the Zion Christian Church in high numbers in search of what Anderson (2001) calls 'prophetic healing'.

The growth of the Zion Christian Church has something to do with the healing practices through the ritual healing process. In other words, unlike in Western Christian churches, the healing practices in this Church involve the use of various symbols and objects. Anderson (2001:111) states, 'The uses of healing symbols is one of the central and most important features of the Church's life, in the South African [context].' The point made here is that healing, particularly the ritual healing processes, plays a major role in attracting Africans to the Zion Christian Church because the people are already used to these practices from an African spiritual perspective. As they are already part of the African spirituality context, these aspects make the church attractive to many Africans on the continent and the diaspora. According to Anderson (2001:107), healing is not just a point of attraction but also the main activity of the church. This means that as opposed to the Western missionary churches, people join churches such as Zion Christian Church not to listen to the sermon but to receive healing in their lives. The prophet in this case is seen as someone who carries the power to heal the sick by praying over the various rituals for healing to happen in the life of the patient. Anderson (2001:113) reiterates the point that these healing practices are what makes Africans, particularly those living in rural areas, join the church in high numbers. However, the Zion Christian Church, as discussed before, is also attractive to Africans in the urban areas, particularly in townships where there is a Zion Christian Church branch. There are branches in almost all the townships in South Africa. Some South Africans also drive from suburban areas to townships for fellowship at the branches of the Zion Christian Church. Therefore, whether in villages or townships, the point made here is that this church is attractive to many adherents, hence its growth across the continent of Africa and the diaspora. The reasons for drawing high numbers can be summarized as the ritual healing process. These factors together with the idea of social isolation and taboos will be discussed in greater detail in the next five chapters to construct a theology of the ritual healing process in African Independent Churches.

Conclusion

This chapter looked at the early developments of the Zion Christian Church (the Star) in Moria, Polokwane, Limpopo province. This church is of high interest in the study of the ritual healing process. The church is relevant for understanding the foundations of the healing practices in the broader scope of the African Independent Churches. Therefore, it was important in this chapter to classify the Zion Christian Church as a Spirit-type African Independent Church with its foundation in the role of the Holy Spirit in prophetic revelation. In addition, this church is founded on the role of the Holy Spirit in the daily activities of the believers. The Zion Church has some influence on the Pentecostal movement through the connection of leaders such as Edward Motaung. In addition, the early development of the Zion Christian Church is also linked to the Zionism of John Alexander Dowie and the beginning of the Zionist movement in South Africa with the influence of leaders such as Daniel Bryant. Thus, the Zion Christian Church is directly linked with the African Zionism movement. The links to Pentecostalism demonstrate that this church has strong Christian foundations which are important in the dissociation of traditional African medicine from the ritual healing process in the Zion Christian Church. About the link with Dowie's Zionism, this should not be mistaken as a direct influence of the West on an African church, as the Zion Christian Church purely remains an African Independent Church without assistance from the West. The chapter also explored the current growth of the Zion Christian Church which makes the church relevant for studying the ritual healing process. Therefore, this church is an important case study for understanding the role of the ritual healing process and its theology in the African Independent Churches.

3

Purification rituals in the Zion Christian Church

Introduction

This chapter identifies different purification rituals in the Zion Christian Church by using the ritual healing theory to trace the origin of healing in this church and its disconnections to traditional African medicine. One of the healing practices in the Zion Christian Church is the use of prayer by the church leader (pastor or minister). But the minister does not use the traditional laying on of hands but rather a piece of wood (*kotana*) and a sheet of paper waved rapidly over the patient's body. In addition, the pastor or the minister in the Zion Christian Church would use the healing practice of the blessed tea, which is also an important aspect of the discussion on dissociating traditional African medicine from ritual healing in this church. The chapter also discusses the use of holy water, which is also prayed over by the pastor or the minister of the Zion Christian Church. Water as a healing practice is also used in conjunction with water baptism. Another healing practice in the Zion Christian Church is pricking using a needle, which is prayed over by the minister in the church and can be applied to the nose, the hands and the legs. This too is pivotal in studying the disconnections of traditional African medicine with ritual healing in the Zion Christian Church. The other healing practice is the use of salted water as a laxative measure for the cleansing of the body and purification. This practice is used to maintain purification in the body by taking out any unwanted substances in the patient's body. Among the children, this is used with the enema for the cleansing and purification of their bodies. The other popular healing practice discussed here is steaming, which is used to deal with headaches or fever for adults and children. The last common healing practice in the Zion Christian Church is the confession of sins, which is believed to be the most important practice that should follow every healing practice and one that is consistent with Christian practices. All these practices are discussed here to highlight the disconnections between traditional African medicine and the ritual healing practices in the Zion Christian Church.

Piece of wood and paper

The Zion Christian Church uses a piece of wood which is known as *kotana* in Northern Sotho as part of the ritual healing process (Anderson 2001:113). The wood is normally applied to the head of the patient as part of healing them. This piece of wood is also used for patting people on their heads for their healing. Lukhaimane (1980:58) cf. Moripe (1996:89) explains that a *kotana*, 'a small piece of wood of about six centimetres long and one-and-a-half centimetres thick', is used to slightly hit [someone] on their body, especially on the painful places. It is believed that patting with the wood would bring healing because this wood has been prayed for and blessed by the bishop. This means that this piece of wood is not limited to the head of the patient but can be applied to the shoulders, the feet and other parts of the body. It also means that it is the responsibility of the patient to explain to the minister where the pain is located so that the piece of wood can be applied correctly. The use of a piece of wood as it is done in the Zion Christian Church falls within the framework of the use of plants within the ritual healing process (Sofowora 1996). Bird (2024:86) explains that within the ritual healing process, holding a piece of wood in your hand demonstrates a form of energy that the healer possesses against diseases. This piece of wood produces a certain energy from the healer towards the sickness and the disease of the individual. While scholars such as Sundkler (1961), Hanekom (1975) and Mokgobi (2014) associate practices such as the holding of a piece of wood in the Zion Christian Church with traditional African medicine, I argue here that its use should be separated from that of the traditional healer as prayer is a priority to the wood.

The Zion Christian Church also uses a piece of paper that is waved on the patient while saying some prayers for the patient (Anderson 2001:113). This kind of paper is used in the Zion Christian Church as part of the ritual healing process. The papers are usually cut from the newspapers and blessed by the ministers to effect healing upon the sick bodies. Lukhaimane (1980:57) explains that when the Zion Christian Church started in the first quarter of the twentieth century, they used pieces of khaki cloth as a healing practice; however, as the church grew in large numbers, this became an expensive exercise. Hence, the church started using pieces of newspaper. The piece of khaki corresponded with the colours of the church, particularly those of the male choir also known as *mokhukhu*. However, as explained by Lukhaimane (1980), this became a very expensive exercise for the church; hence, they resorted to the use of newspaper which became readily available. This means that the ministers of the church are required to gather the pieces of the newspaper every week in the fulfilment of the healing practice of the use of papers in the Zion Christian Church. The ministers and the pastors also must bless the same papers so that they become blessed to be used in the ritual healing process. Once prayed over by the bishop or the ministers, these would no longer become ordinary newspapers but blessed ones that can be used as purification rituals in the church. In the Zion Christian Church, the papers are not only waved to the patient but there is also a practice of patting the same papers on the body of the patient to invoke healing upon them. This again should be distinguished from the use of papers in traditional African medicine which would invoke spirits whilst waving or burning papers. Horton (1967) adds that in traditional African medicine, they would also be calling names of people while using papers which is not something done at the Zion Christian Church.

Another healing practice in the Zion Christian Church is the burning of a paper and waving it around the head of the patient to demonstrate that this is fire around them (Anderson 1999:301). So, the newspapers which are collected by the ministers are cut and burnt to be waived around the heads of the patients. Daneel (2019:44) explains that the burning of paper in which the patient inhales the smoke coming out of it corresponds very well with the burning of incense in traditional African medicine. I would argue that there are distinctions between the burning of incense within the African traditional healing process done by the traditional healer and the burning of a paper in the Zion Christian Church. Within African Traditional religions, the burning of incense is important beyond the process of healing as it also serves as part of ancestral worship. Staub, Geck and Weckerle (2011) explain that the burning of incense is a communicative tool through which people speak to their ancestors. However, burning fire around the patients in the Zion Christian Church symbolizes the fire of God as was the case in the Old Testament as a sign that God protects his people against evil attack by the evil one. God promised his children that he would not remove the pillar of cloud by day and the pillar of fire by night (exodus 13:21). In other African Independent Churches, there would be a burning of candles as part of a healing practice and a form of protection for the patients or simply a way of making prayers to

God. The burning of candles is also used as a symbol of the protection of God upon his people, not necessarily the worship of ancestors as done in African traditional religions. Therefore, the burning of incense and the burning of papers as used in the Zion Christian Church corresponds very well with the Old Testament practice but should be distinguished from the practices in the African Traditional religions. It must be understood in the context of a ritual healing process as Abrams (2021:174) concludes that 'burning sacred herbs, barks, and resins has always been a part of ritual healing process across the continent and diaspora'. I have observed over the years ministers in the Zion Christian Church burning papers; however, there would be no corresponding action that demonstrates that it is connected with ancestral worship.

Blessed tea

The Zion Christian Church uses tea and coffee that has been manufactured in the church as part of the ritual healing purposes (Anderson 2001:112). The use of tea as a purification ritual is mainly for the purification of the body and the deliverance of the patient from evil spirits (Go 2016:254). The tea in this church is very popular, and it is known as the tea that gives life to the patient, also known as *tee ya bophelo* in Northern Sotho. This implies that upon taking the tea, the patient would receive life, and the sickness and disease would disappear as the tea gives life. It is believed that after taking such a tea, the sick person would be given life, and the sickness would disappear in their life. Anderson (2001:112) gives an example of a 'child [that] had been healed of a deformity after the child had been given this tea together with water from a spring'. Therefore, tea, unlike other forms of healing practices within the ritual healing process in the Zion Christian Church, can be prescribed to children and not just adults alone. In addition, the tea made in the Zion Christian Church is not only used for drinking to bring purification but also during bathing by the patients. Therefore, the members of the Zion Christian Church would mix tea and coffee with the bathing water as part of the purification ritual in the church. The tea in the Zion Christian Church is popularly known as *tee ya thapelo*, which is directly interpreted as the tea of prayer. Mashabela (2017:6) points out that it is this aspect of prayer in the use of tea that brings connections between ritual healing and Christian practices. Again we see connections between a healing ritual and a Christian spiritual discipline such as prayer. This is not the case in traditional African medicine.

Lukhaimane (1980:105) explains that tea as a ritual healing practice in the Zion Christian Church corresponds well with herbal tea or what others call bush tea (Rakuambo et al. 2009). Mahomoodally (2013) mentions *Cyclopia genistoides* which is 'an indigenous herbal tea to South Africa and considered as a health food. Traditionally, the leafy shoots and flowers were fermented and dried to prepare tea. It has also been used since early times for its direct positive effects on the urinary system and is valued as a stomachic that aids weak digestion without affecting the heart.' This means that in the use of tea the Zion Christian Church is helping its members indigenously to fight against many forms of sicknesses and diseases. Joubert et al. (2008:376) mention the *Athrixia* whose functions 'include treatment of boils, acne, infected wounds, and infected throats'. Another tea *Aspalathus linearis* is popularly known as 'Rooibos' in South Africa and has enjoyed commercial success. Joubert et al. (2008:376) explain,

> Rooibos tea was considered healthy, based on the fact that it was 'harmless and satisfying' due to the absence of alkaloids and a low tannin content. It was only after the discovery by Annetjie Theron in 1968 that an infusion of rooibos, when administered to her colicky baby, cured the chronic restlessness, vomiting, and stomach cramps, that rooibos became well-known as a 'healthy' beverage, leading to a broader consumer base. Many babies since have been reared with rooibos either added to their milk, or given as a weak brew. Anecdotal evidence suggests that it has an anti-allergic effect, improves appetite, reduces nervous tension, and promotes sound sleep. It also alleviates ingestion, heartburn, and nausea. Topical applications of rooibos extract are believed to alleviate dermatological problems, i.e. eczema, acne, and nappy rash.

It appears to me that the leadership of the Zion Christian Church might have had prior knowledge of the importance of all these different types of tea in the health of their members. Hence, there is the use of tea as a purification ritual not necessarily as a traditional African medicine.

The Zion Christian Church uses a special tea called *tee ya senepe*, which is directly translated as the 'tea of the photo' which means the tea bearing the photograph of the bishop. This tea is special since it carries the photo of the bishop, and it means it is already blessed even before the bishop or any other minister can start praying for it. The tea in Moria is different from the ordinary tea that one buys from the shop. Therefore, the followers of the Zion Christian Church would prefer this tea unless the prophet prescribed other forms of tea or a popular tea or coffee. However, even when other forms of tea are prescribed, the members would still mix them with the tea from Moria or the one bearing the photo of the bishop. It is not only the tea that bears the photo of the bishop, but members would also have big pictures with the photo of Engenas Lekganyane, Edward Lekganyane and the current bishop, Barnabas Lekganyane. These are used not only as healing practices but also as protective practices as will be discussed in the next chapter of this book. What is important in this section is that tea is ordinarily used as a purification ritual without necessarily linking it with traditional African medicine. The reason for this assertion is that even non-believers or non-religious people use tea for purification and health reasons.

The members of the church have the propensity to come to the church early so that they can receive the tea before the start of the service. In evening services where the church starts late, it is a propensity of the church members to first start by drinking tea in preparation for the service. The men who joined the male choir (*mokhukhu*) would also drink tea in preparation for singing and dancing in the night. It is perceived that this tea is the one that gives men energy to dance throughout the night. It is, therefore, very common in the Zion Christian Church to see men sitting together drinking tea in cups. Even in ceremonies such as *mpoho* (prayer night), which is supposed to last for the whole night, what keeps the members going is the drinking of the tea which not only brings healing but is also more like an energy booster. Therefore, Lukhaimane (1980) highlighted above that tea encourages fellowship in the Zion Christian Church. But more than its *koinonia* functions, it brings healing, energy and strength to the adherents of the Zion Christian Church. For men, the tea is made stronger and sometimes mixed with coffee and with a bit of cooking oil; hence, they can dance throughout the night during the *mokhukhu*, the male choir dance. This section was aimed at highlighting the use of tea as a purification ritual, and it was found that indeed tea comes from different medicinal plants in South Africa and elsewhere in the world. However, there is no connection between the use of tea in the Zion Christian Church and tea in traditional African medicine. On the contrary, it was found that tea is used by ordinary men and women who seek purification and health in their lives.

Holy water

The Zion Christian Church uses water that the minister prays over as part of the ritual healing process. A popular practice in the church is the sprinkling of water on the patient three times on their face and under their feet to invoke healing. The minister would also sprinkle water on the back of an individual in need of healing with great force. This water is meant to bring healing to the patient, particularly when it is prayed over by the minister or the pastor of the church. There is also a practice of sprinkling water upon the adherents of the church each time they come to a spiritual service for their purification. This means that there is no way that an adherent of the Zion Christian Church can enter the church premises without being sprinkled water upon. This is done to ensure that the members of the church are delivered from evil forces before they can enter the church premises. Other than sprinkling water on individuals, the minister can decide to splash a large quantity onto the audience. I have observed over the years that this is also done to ensure that the members of the church are awake for the duration of the church service. It is a propensity of the church members to fall asleep, particularly during ceremonies such as *mpoho* (the night prayer). Thus, splashing water is not only a ritual healing practice but also a measure that helps the congregants stay awake during the night service. Under this gesture, it is seldom that the congregants would wipe such water off their faces as they believe that this too is a sign that they are blessed, and they have been prayed for by the church minister or pastor.

The bishop or a minister would bless the water, hence the concept of the blessed holy water as opposed to carrying ordinary water. However, the holy water is not always prayed over by the minister as the church members can pray over the water as well (Anderson 2001:113). The members are always required to follow some rituals such as women covering their heads and men wearing jackets to ensure that the water is blessed. In addition, this is also observed when receiving water from the ministers. Similarly, when women receive prayers for the blessed water, they need to cover their heads, and for men who are receiving prayers, they should wear a jacket for the prayers or the blessed water to work. According to Daneel (2019:19), it is also common among the followers of the Zion Christian Church to bring bottles of water to be blessed so that when the time of sickness comes, they can use the same water on their own. Therefore, it is a propensity of the followers of the Zion Christian Church to carry bottles of water and sometimes even buckets of water when going to church, as it serves as an opportunity to receive blessings and prayers from the ministers and the pastors. The water from the rivers and streams is perceived as carrying more healing powers and blessings than the normal water from the tap. The use of natural water from streams and wells is part of a ritual healing process.

Water as a purification ritual is also used by offering it to congregants to drink for them to heal from illness. Thus, it is not only sprinkled or splashed on the bodies of the adherents of the Zion Christian Church, but they should also drink it. Hence, after sprinkling it on the body of the patient, it is also given to the individual to drink. There are some patriarchal practices on serving the blessed water to the congregants as the purification ritual. I remember that when the pastors prayed for us, as men, we would remain standing, but for women, they would either bend a bit or kneel as a sign of humility and a gesture to receive the blessings. However, this should not be seen as patriarchal practices but rather gestures of humility and submission which are all part of a ritual healing process.

There is also the drinking of boiled warm water called *mogabulo*, which is another purification ritual in the Zion Christian Church. The church minister, like in all other purification rituals in the Zion Christian Church, is responsible for the blessing of the boiled warm water. *Mogabulo* is very popular in the Zion Christian Church and is normally used by many followers as a purification ritual. According to Lukhaimane (1980:58), the members of the church would drink *mogabulo* in the early hours of the morning and late in the evening. However, Wouters (2014:119) explains that *mogabulo* is not just ordinary boiled water but is normally boiled in specially prepared water in the open air and often in a 20 litre tin, which after being heated would be served to the patients. This healing practice again is very much connected to the ritual healing process, particularly in how the boiled water is prepared for the patients. Thus, it is not a simple practice where one can just drink warm water from the kettle; rather, it needs to be prepared by adhering to specific rituals within the Zion Christian Church. The use of boiled water as a purification ritual is perceived as a substance giving life to the patients.

Generally, water in the Zion Christian Church and other African Independent Churches is used as a purification substance (Anderson 2001:112). Daneel (2019:19) concurs that '[t]his blessed water is later used for purification purposes, exorcism, and medicinal treatment'. Hence, other than the water used by the minister, the members can have the water that they will use in their houses. It is believed in the Zion Christian Church that water serves as purification in the same way as it did in the Old Testament. Anderson (2001:112) explains:

> The use of this water is justified from a biblical point of view by reference to God's promise to cleanse his people from all their impurities by the sprinkling of clean water (Ezekiel 36:25); the practice in the Torah of sprinkling water on a person polluted by contact with a corpse (Numbers 19:11–12); and the fact that the Spirit of God hovered' over the waters (Genesis 1:1). It is therefore believed that the Holy Spirit is present in water that has been blessed or in the water of the river of baptism.

Moripe (1996:87) agrees with the connection of water and Spirit when he says that 'Spirit, breath, and water are all seen as essentially animating; they are substantial yet fluid, containable yet self-regulating, and they are capable of pervading space within and outside the body. The Zionist churches are sometimes referred to as Didiba (wells).' Nonetheless, it should be reiterated that water is mainly used for purification. It is for the same reasons that the members of the Zion Christian Church believe that they should be sprinkled with water after attending a funeral for cleansing. In addition, they would also wash in the blessed water after attending a funeral or immediately after coming from the graveyard.

Some scholars connect the use of water in the Zion Christian Church with traditional African medicine. One such scholar is Lukhaimane (1980:58), who opined that '[t]he origin of sprinkling people with water as a means to purify them is also found in African tradition. In many communities, especially of the Sotho group, water is used to sprinkle on people after a funeral.' However, we cannot connect traditional African medicine with the use of water in the Zion Christian Church just because they both use water. Even Sundkler (1961:232) acknowledged that most Zionist churches pray for the water to be blessed before they can give it to the patients. This has nothing to do with traditional African medicine. While I agree with Mokgobi (2014:6) that African Independent Churches do use water, I differ with him when he connects the use of water in this religious group with ancestral worship. After all, every human being on earth uses water. There are no variables that support the connection of the use of water in the Zion Christian Church with that of traditional African medicine. Therefore, water like many other purification rituals in this chapter should be seen as part of the ritual healing process within the Zion Christian Church. Mashabela (2017:7) quotes Lebeloane and Madise (2006) who concurs that within the context of the ritual healing process, 'water is perceived as a gift from the Creator. It is further understood to have life-giving and life-invigorating power if it has been blessed by a minister of religion.' Therefore, water is the source of life and an important commodity in human life. However, water is more important to the ministers in African Independent Churches like the Zion Christian Church.

Water baptism

Water baptism is a common practice in the Christian tradition which serves as a sacrament demonstrating the death and resurrection of Christ. The

Zion Christian Church as per the vision that the founding father, Engenas Lekganyane, received in 1910 baptizes in three-times immersion or simply triple immersion. As discussed in the previous chapter, triple immersion is a common practice among the classical Pentecostal churches such as the Apostolic Faith Mission of South Africa. Hence, this method of baptism is also something that makes the connections between early Pentecostalism and the Zion Christian Church very strong. However, the difference between early Pentecostalism and the Zion Christian Church is the location of baptism. Like many other African Independent Churches, the Zion Christian Church baptizes its members in the running water based on their understanding of baptism as something to be done in the water that is in motion. Moripe (1996:49) explains, 'There is a river, running through Moria, and it is called Kwenane, and it is where "Believers Baptism" takes place.' In addition, this is because the Zion Christian Church believes that the baptism should be done in living water of a large quantity (Lukhaimane 1980:46). In this way, running water like the one in the river is considered living water also containing a lot of water. It is for this reason that other forms of baptism such as sprinkling water on the forehead are not accepted as baptism methods in the Zion Christian Church. Therefore even in baptism, the Zion Christian Church does not follow the Western paradigms in coloniality but the African paradigms in decoloniality. It is also expected that with the water baptism practice, there will also follow the baptism in the Holy Spirit whereby all those who are baptized in water will receive the Holy Spirit (Lukhaimane 1980:91). The latter is also a strong connection with early Pentecostalism as there is an emphasis on the baptism of the Holy Spirit accompanied by the baptism in water as was the case when Jesus was baptized in the Jordan River. Therefore, the water baptism in the Zion Christian Church has some form of parallelism with the baptism in classical Pentecostal churches in the way it is done and with its connection with the baptism in the Holy Spirit. Water baptism disconnects with traditional African medicine such that even Sundkler (1961:225), a critic of African Independent Churches, acknowledged that baptism is used to purify those who have been made unclean.

But there are some differences as well. Whereas water baptism in classical Pentecostal churches such as the Apostolic Faith Mission symbolizes the death and the resurrection of Christ, water baptism in the Zion Christian Church is considered a ritual healing practice. The reason is that through baptism every form of uncleanness including diseases is expected to leave the one who is being baptized. The use of baptism as a healing practice is further explained by the leadership of the Zion Christian Church quoted in Lukhaimane (1980:48) where

Edward Lekganyane said: 'Baptism was like dipping cattle to remove ticks or skin diseases. They should be submerged in water and not be sprinkled. The new converts, he continued, were like these cattle, they had to be completely submerged in the water.' Thus, by connecting baptism with cattle dipping, the bishop is moving away from the traditional meaning of baptism to locate it within the ritual healing process. This is the same reason that baptism in the Zion Christian Church is practised in its full nature, not forehead baptism or sprinkling baptism or anything like that as discussed above. Therefore, when immersing the congregants three times in water, it is expected that diseases would leave them the same way when the cattle go through the dipping process. However, this does not mean that baptism in the Zion Christian Church is reserved for the sick, but it does mean that anyone who is sick gets healed upon taking part in the baptismal ritual. Besides, even those who may consider themselves as not sick in the physical sense might be sick spiritually as per the definition of sickness in the Zion Christian Church. Therefore, baptism is considered a healing practice for not only those who are sick in their bodies but also those who are sick spiritually. The goal is to remove any form of evil, uncleanness, impurity and any other impediments during the baptism healing practice. Hence, followers of the Zion Christian Church look forward to the baptism ceremony for these benefits and to obtain membership in the church.

Water baptism is considered a healing practice because there is also a tendency to conduct other purification rituals before the ceremony of the baptism. The believers who are supposed to be baptized are required to confess their sins to the minister or the pastor even before baptism. In addition, other purification rituals such as pricking and vomiting can take place leading up to the baptism practice. Lukhaimane (1980:47) points out that 'if the convert was a medicine person, he or she was asked to hand over all his or her "tools" which were then burnt in public'. Therefore, in the Zion Christian Church and other Zionist churches, baptism is more than a religious rite and is performed beyond its sacramental meaning of death and resurrection of Christ to also serve as a ritual healing practice. It is also correct to point out that baptism in the Zion Christian Church is considered a purification ritual more than symbolizing the forgiveness of sins. In traditional African medicine, the concept of washing in water is also performed for healing or delivering the patient. This is because, within traditional African medicine, it is believed that the various spirits that are tormenting people can be released into the water when delivering a patient. It is for this reason that scholars such as Sundkler (1961) and Mokgobi (2014) would connect the use of water in traditional African medicine and water in ritual healing in the Zion Christian Church. However, these scholars fail to understand that water in the Zion Christian Church is in conjunction with the Christian faith and sacrament whereas, in traditional African medicine, water is used in connection with marine spirits. Therefore, as much as both use water, there are serious disconnections in the rationale behind the usage.

Pricking

The other healing practice that is used in the Zion Christian Church is pricking the human body to invoke the release of blood. This is known as *go phula madi* in Northern Sotho. According to Anderson (2001:113 cf 1999:307), 'for this process, a prophet prescribes exactly where a patient should be pricked on the hands, legs or in the nostrils to get rid of "impure blood", which is traditionally believed to be the source of sickness and pain'. Daneel (2019:46) concurs that pricking is done for the removal of evil blood from the life of a patient which could in a way have caused the disease in the first place. Pricking in the Zion Christian Church is also done to deal with abnormal growths in the body in the same way the medical doctors would do when dealing with growths in their patients. Akyeampong and Gates (2012:485) point out that pricking is one of the important healing practices in the Zion Christian Church because during the process all unwanted blood that causes diseases is removed from the patient. The prophet will prescribe this healing practice if they consider the unwanted blood to be the primary causative factor to the disease suffered by the patient. Grant and Mansell (2008:448) add that it is a healing practice in the Zion Christian Church designed to specifically remove the pain in addition to other purification rituals that bring healing. Nthabu (1989:68) concurs that pricking by a needle which is blessed by the bishop is important for the removal of impure blood in sensitive areas such as the eye and the arteries. Therefore, when applying pricking as the healing practice, the Zion Christian Church aims to deal with all the diseases that are caused by impure blood. Hence, pricking as a purification ritual was applied to elderly people who have blood-related diseases (Lukhaimane 1980:58). I can attest to this fact because as a follower of this church for many years, I have not seen a child being pricked through a needle but only adults, particularly the elderly people.

It must be reiterated that pricking is not done with an ordinary needle but with a special one that has been prayed over by the bishop (Lukhaimane 1980:58). In addition, it is also important to point out that this is such a very sensitive purification ritual, and as such it was not done randomly but as per the instructions of the prophet (Lukhaimane 1980:58). Moripe (1996:103) explains the processes in which pricking is conducted at the Zion Christian Church:

> The needles shall then be put into a pot of boiling water and left to boil for 10 to 15 minutes; After they have boiled for 10 to 15 minutes, the needles shall then be removed from the pot and allowed to cool down, until they are cold; Then the minister bathes the legs and/fore-arms of the patient with the holy water; Then the minister uses the needle on the patient; When the minister has finished with the particular patient, the needle which he was using on that patient is washed with the holy water, and returned to the pot of boiling water; the needle must again be allowed to boil for 10 to 15 minutes before it is removed from the pot and allowed to cool down. It can now be used again.

This process as explained by Moripe (1996:103) ensures that the needle remains healthy before it is used for the next person. It is also done so that pricking as a purification ritual is connected to other purification rituals like the blessed water or the holy water in this regard. This procedure according to Moripe (1996:103) was also prescribed by the bishop to avoid infection of HIV-AIDS from one patient to the other because of the possible sharing of blood during pricking. This means that the bishop and the Zion Christian Church are aware that if the needle is not cleaned, it can cause disease for the next patient.

Some scholars make connections between pricking in the Zion Christian Church and traditional African medicine such as Lukhaimane (1980:58) who said,

> Traditionally, impure blood was regarded as a source of pain, headache, eye disease, or many other bodily pains. To remove impure blood medicine men used to cut an artery or cut a person on his joints or anywhere where there was pain. Some would [apply] a method of sucking out blood [from] their patients.

This process as described by Lukhaimane (1980) is called 'cupping' where the healer cuts out certain flesh in the body and sucks out the blood to remove the unwanted blood from the patient. This ensures that the pain is removed from the patient for them to receive healing. Turner (1992:192) explains that in traditional African medicine, the healer would identify where the pain is and cut out the flesh to remove the pain from the body. This process is similar to the pricking of the needle in the Zion Christian Church as they both aim to remove unwanted blood from the life of the patient. This is important in traditional African medicine and the Zion Christian Church to deal with chronic diseases, particularly those caused by unwanted blood. Cupping according to

Onwueme (2014:7) is a blood-letting process that is also used for the removal of unwanted blood:

> It was administered as a cure for a wide range of ailments, especially backache and headache. The tool for the process was a long hollow gourd that was tapered at one end, giving a funnel-like conical shape. Incisions were made on the patient with a razor. Then the wide part of the gourd was placed over the wound. The healer then administered mouth suction through the narrow part of the gourd. This created a vacuum that increased the outward flow of 'bad' blood into the base of the gourd. When sucking stopped, the vacuum was maintained for several additional minutes by placing a supple piece of leaf over the narrow end of the gourd. At the end of the process, the clump of congealed 'bad' blood at the wide base of the gourd was discarded, and healing concoctions were rubbed into the wound.

Hence, it is common to find the body of an ordinary African with many marks of razors as they have been cupped to deal with unwanted blood in their body and apply healing through the use of concoctions. However, I would still argue here that even though both traditional African medicine and the Zion Christian Church engage in the process of removing unwanted blood, it does not mean that the church has borrowed this method from the traditional African religions. I would rather classify this method as an indigenous practice than a traditional African medicine practice.

Salted water

The salted water (known as *meetse a letswai* in Northern Sotho) is a purification practice in the Zion Christian Church used as a laxative for the cleansing of the body. The patients, particularly adults, are normally instructed by prophets to drink this salted water which becomes a laxative for the cleansing of the body, specifically the digestive system. This purification ritual is particularly used for the evacuation of the stool to avoid complications in the stomach and related diseases. The salt that is normally used is called *letswai la croft*, which simply means the croft salt which can also be purchased at the headquarters of the church in Moria, Boyne. The croft salt is normally added to the boiling water to produce the salted water for cleansing. The patient would normally wake up early in the morning to drink this salted water and be engaged in the cleansing process throughout the day. During this ritual process, the patient is required not to eat anything; otherwise, it would interfere with the whole process of cleansing. This means that the drinking of salted water in the Zion Christian Church is somehow related to fasting in the Christian tradition. However, in classical Pentecostal churches such as the Apostolic Faith Mission of South Africa, fasting is not combined with other practices such as the drinking of salted water. In the latter, fasting would just mean the abstinence of food for a day or more for prayer. However, in the Zion Christian Church, the members would target weekends for the drinking of salted water to cleanse the digestive system.

In addition, the salted water is also used to induce vomiting which is called *o kapa* in Northern Sotho. So, after drinking a lot of salted water, the patient in the Zion Christian Church would use their index finger to touch their uvula so that they could induce vomiting. Lukhaimane (1980:49) explains that vomiting was the process of releasing the excess bile from the body of the patient. It is believed that during vomiting all the unwanted objects inside the stomach of the patient would be removed and the patient would receive healing (Anderson 1999:300). However, the process of vomiting is not only used for the removal of the physical objects but also the spiritual defilement that caused sickness in the first place. Therefore, once the prophet discovers that the body of the patient is defiled, they would recommend vomiting using salted water. The patient can apply this water alone without the supervision of the prophet or the church minister. Vomiting as part of cleansing is a lot more common in traditional African medicine. It is common in traditional African medicine to prescribe vomiting to their patient to heal or deliver them. Rio, MacCarthy and Blanes (2017:136) explain that 'vomiting and physical extraction are unsurprisingly some of the more common purifying practices'. Although this practice is not so common in classical Pentecostal churches, it is also common in neo-Pentecostal churches where members of the church are expected to vomit some substances during healing and deliverance. Therefore, by vomiting, the patient can be sure that their healing and deliverance have come. Therefore, vomiting is not unique to the ritual healing process in the Zion Christian Church but is practised elsewhere even by neo-Pentecostals. However, the fact that it is practised by most religious groups does not mean that there is a connection between the ritual healing process in the Zion Christian Church and traditional African medicine. While scholars such as Sundkler (1961:22) have connected the vomiting of traditional healers with vomiting as a healing ritual in African Independent Churches, I would caution against this position as it all depends on how these methods are applied by each religious group.

The same salted water as a purification ritual in the Zion Christian Church is used among children through an enema which is inserted in their bums also for cleansing. Similarly, the children are required not to eat anything during that time when the parents would be using an enema on their bodies. This is to ensure that the ritual healing process is effective as a cleansing method for the children. Once the enema is applied onto their bodies, the children would be engaged in a cleansing process where every unwanted object in their bodies would be removed. This is important during the school holidays particularly in the festive seasons during Christmas or even Easter when the children have been eating a lot. The enema would then be used to cleanse them which maintains the healthy standard in their bodies. The use of an enema among children is a common ritual healing process. This method is also used to help children deal with constipation; hence, it has been a common ritual healing process. The mistake that scholars such as Sundkler (1961:233) make is to link this practice in the Zion Christian Church and traditional African medicine. According to Sundkler (1961:233), the Zion Christian Church in the use of enema has learned from traditional African medicine. Sundkler (1961:233) says that it is common for the prophets in the Zionist churches to carry the enema syringe around their neck for purification among their members of followers as a practice that they have learned from the traditional African religions. However, I would argue that the Zion Christian Church is using this practice as part of ritual healing practice and not necessarily borrowing from traditional African medicine.

However, it seems like the purification ritual using salted water as a laxative for vomiting and in the enema for children is becoming less popular. As modern medicine has become popular, the use of salted water for cleansing and purification is no longer popular, even among the adherents of the Zion Christian Church. Lukhaimane (1980:77) explains that 'the use of salt for cleaning the bowels as [ritual healing method] is gradually giving way in favour of the medical treatment in clinics and hospitals'. This is even more immanent in the twenty-first century than in the twentieth century when Lukhaimane did his fieldwork in the Zion Christian Church. This means that as modern laxatives are introduced as a cleansing method in clinics and hospitals, the use of salted water is becoming less and less popular even among the followers of the Zion Christian Church. However, the point being made here is that this purification ritual should not be confused with its practices in traditional African medicine as scholars such as Sundkler (1961) and Lukhaimane (1980) have done.

Steaming

Steaming is another purification ritual used in the Zion Christian Church, which is known as *go arabela* in Northern Sotho. This purification ritual is used to deal with headaches and fever among both adults and children by purifying the body through sweating. This ritual healing process is done by fetching stones from the mountain which are burned in the fire and put inside the boiling water to produce the steam. The patient is then asked to cover themselves with boiling water combined with stones for a few minutes to steam their body. Steaming is done under the supervision of the minister in the Zion Christian Church or simply the elder in the household with experience. However, whoever is conducting this ritual healing process is supposed to put on a jacket for the process to work in the life of the patient. The prophet would prescribe the use of steam as a purification ritual to the patient. In giving this instruction, the prophet would outline a specific mountain from which the patient can obtain the stones to use together with boiled water. Steaming as a purification ritual according to Bird (2022:151) is used for the detoxification of the person as a whole, that is, the body, the mind and the spirit. Bird (2010) points out that steaming has been part of the ritual healing process together with bathing and other rituals. It has been an important purification ritual in helping patients to heal fever and flu through sweating. Carrasco et al. (2019:59) add, 'Steaming in its current form is used to treat conditions believed to have spiritual causes. Steaming allows the body to be cleansed and rid of impurities. Through steaming, the body opens to absorb the medicine selected to treat the cause of the problems.' But I would argue again that in practicing steaming as part of a ritual healing process, the Zion Christian Church does not necessarily borrow from the traditional African religions but rather from the indigenous knowledge systems in Africa.

The confession of sins and faith

The last, but not least, purification ritual in the Zion Christian Church is the confession of sins, which is believed to be the most important practice that should follow every healing practice in the church. In this way, confession in the Zion Christian Church is also considered a purification ritual encompassing a whole range of other healing practices. In other words, it is believed that nothing would happen until one confesses their sins to receive their healing (Anderson 2001:113). The confession of sins as part of the ritual healing process is consistent with the biblical texts, for example, in James 5 whereby the sick are encouraged to confess their sins in addition to other healing practices like anointing with oil and prayer. James 5:16 states this very well: 'Therefore confess your sins to each other and pray for each other so that you may be healed. The prayer of a righteous person is powerful and effective.' It is something that is not common in traditional African medicine but in Christianity. Thus, again we see the Zion Christian Church leaning towards the Christian practices of healing rather than traditional African medicine practices. However, in the classical Pentecostal churches, the forgiveness of sins is not done as a purification ritual but as part of salvation. Once saved, the believer is expected to live a holy life. Whereas in the Zion Christian Church, it is expected that the believer even though saved might end up in sin which might hinder their healing, hence the importance of constant confession as part of purification.

The confession of sins is therapeutic in the sense that there are some sicknesses or diseases that are considered to have been caused by unforgiveness and anger. The Zion Christian Church is aware that even though the sickness might manifest in the physical causing some discomfort in the body, it might be symptomatic of unforgiveness. Therefore, according to Moripe (1996), when the patient confesses their sin, they open an opportunity to receive their healing. The minister who is listening to the patient's confessions must have the ability to sympathize with the patient. Moripe (1996:104) continues to say that this purification ritual 'consists in feeling with that person's psyche. It's a deep respect for the facts of the man who suffers from them and for the riddle of such a man's life an unprejudiced objectivity.' Therefore, the minister, pastor or even a prophet in the Zion Christian Church is expected to have the ability to listen to the confessions of the patient without prejudice. The main aim is to lead the patient to the forgiveness of sins rather than becoming too judgmental of what they have done in the past. Therefore, the confession of sins within the healing process is necessary as the cause of sickness is not only physical but also psychological and spiritual requiring the intervention through confession of sins. It is also important to point out that in the Zion Christian Church, this is also important in ensuring that the other purification rituals such as pricking, holy water, the use of paper, the use of wood, steaming, the use of salted water and others become effective in helping out the patient.

The confession of sins is supposed to be done to the church minister or pastor in confidence without the presence of other members of the church. Hence, it is an individualistic act rather than the act of a group or a family. It is known as *go ipolela* in Northern Sotho, which has the implications of individual confession rather than group confession. According to Lukhaimane (1980:45), the ministers during great conferences like Easter are required to attend in large numbers so that they can attend to the issue of listening to confessions of members of the Zion Christian Church because many would be in attendance during these conferences. However, confessing sins is not compulsory or forced in the Zion Christian Church. If a member feels that they do not have anything to confess, they can continue with the other activities within the Zion Christian Church liturgy or even the activities of the conference. However, it would still be emphasized that going through a water baptism ritual and other purification rituals without confession might be dangerous to a member of the Zion Christian Church. This as opposed to healing the patient might lead to being vulnerable to other forms of sickness and misfortunes. In the Christian tradition, the same warning is given, for example, during holy communion where lack of confession might result in negative repercussions. In this way, confession becomes necessary for the follower or the church member to make sure that they avoid the consequences of misfortunes and other evil things happening in their lives.

It should be emphasized therefore that confession of sins together with faith in God makes the other purification rituals to be effective upon the sick person (Lukhaimane 1980:60). Therefore, the patients are asked to exercise their faith in addition to the utilization of different purification rituals. Hence, there is always a teaching around the source of healing as the belief in God rather than the healing practices. Therefore, in applying the confessions of sins as part of the healing process, the Zion Christian Church places the importance of relying on God for healing as opposed to relying on healing rituals. Hence, I argue here through a ritual healing process that the alignment of the church to traditional religions is quite unfortunate as the church is very much aligned on Christian principles such as forgiveness of sins. Even Sundkler (1961:228) did not make a connection between confession and traditional African medicine but rather between sickness and sin when he said, 'The view that healing should normally be preceded by a confession of sin implies a connexion between sickness and sin.' Again this proves the connection between the Christian faith and the practices of healing in the Zion Christian Church in South Africa.

Conclusion

This chapter discussed the purification rituals in the Zion Christian Church. The main aim of the chapter was to disconnect these rituals from traditional

African medicine. A small piece of wood called *kotana* together with a piece of paper is used in healing rituals in the Zion Christian Church. The study found that the use of wood is part of the use of plants in the ritual healing process. The blessed tea is another purification ritual used by the sick, and the study found that there is some correspondence between the use of tea and the use of other teas in indigenous plants. Holy water, which is normally prayed over by the church minister, is a common purification ritual in the Zion Christian Church. In addition, the church members would be instructed to fetch running water from streams or rivers, which could be brought to be blessed by the church minister. Another purification ritual in the Zion Christian Church is pricking, which is used to reduce the blood levels in the body by using the church needle to take out blood from the patient. The study found that, generally, the shedding of blood is a common practice in traditional African medicine, which also includes pricking or just cutting human beings' flesh through the use of razors. However, we need to observe the differences in the rationale behind the usage of the purification rituals. Salted water as a healing ritual is used as a laxative by drinking it for the cleansing and purification of the patient. The salted water is used among adults to induce vomiting, particularly to deal with the excess of bile. It is also used with the enema, particularly among children for the evacuation of the stool. The study found that the Zion Christian Church does not borrow from traditional African medicine but indigenous knowledge in these practices. Another purification ritual is steaming, which is a common healing practice used even for the healing of both children and the elderly. However, these healing practices in the Zion Christian Church should be differentiated from their practices in the African traditional religions. One such difference is that the Zion Christian Church also uses the confession of sins as a purification ritual, which is believed to be the most important practice that should follow every healing practice. The confession of sins is important in the Zion Christian Church in conscientizing their members about the reliance on God for healing as opposed to the healing practices. Therefore, in most of these practices, there is a clear disconnection between traditional African medicine and the ritual healing practice in the Zion Christian Church.

4

Protection rituals in the Zion Christian Church

Introduction

This chapter discusses the various symbols and practices of protection in the Zion Christian Church. These are used as it is believed that they would be able to bring protection upon the members of the church and also to prevent illnesses and diseases. Church uniform (*seaparo*) is not worn only for the sake of looking good to other church members but also serves as a protective measure against attacks of sickness and diseases. The members and followers of the Zion Christian Church often are instructed to call the church minister to sprinkle water that is mixed with sand for the protection of the household. The members of the church upon receiving baptism in water would be required to wear a badge on their clothes which should be visible to anyone they meet to serve as a protective practice. Another protective healing practice in the Zion Christian Church which is discussed in this chapter is the photograph of the bishop which is popularly known as *senepe sa mookamedi* in Northern Sotho. The members of the church are given the strings and strips to wear around their waist which is known as *motlamo* in Northern Sotho. Attached to the white strings or strips is the blue piece of cloth which is known as *khutane* in Northern Sotho and which is also used for the protection of the believers against assaults and lightning. The members of the Zion Christian Church also use what is known as the brown paper to protect them against non-members, particularly during visitations. The chapter discusses the copper wires known as *mathale* in Northern Sotho that the Zion Christian Church members place around the gates of their houses as a means of protecting them from witchcraft. The male members of the Zion Christian Church use the sticks known as *dipatla* also for protection against any attack from enemies. The church's male members, particularly during their *mokhukhu* (male choir) sessions, would carry the whip known as *sefepi* in

Northern Sotho, which they use for protection. We discuss these practices here in our quest to understand the protective systems in the Zion Christian Church, which have implications for healing practices. In other words, in protecting members of the church against diseases and sickness, these protective practices have implications for the ritual healing process.

The wearing of church uniform

The Zion Christian Church, like all other African Independent Churches, believes in the wearing of uniforms. The wearing of the church uniform which is *seaparo sa kereke* in Northern Sotho is one of the protective measures in the Zion Christian Church. Hence, immediately after baptism, the member of the church is required to purchase a uniform. It is important to point out that only baptized members of the church can wear a church uniform (Anderson 2000:158). This includes the children whose parents are full-time members of the church; they too would be allowed to wear the uniform. It is therefore common to see young boys of the baptized members wearing the male uniform. It is a requirement at the Zion Christian Church for the members to either wear a uniform or put on an appropriate dress code which is normally a jacket for men and covering of the head and long dresses for women. However, most of the church members would endeavour to purchase a church uniform to be complete members of the church. If an individual is not dressed appropriately, they would be asked to return home and put on the proper dress code. Again, for those who are wearing their church uniform, this would not be an issue. This practice is common as part of the ritual healing process in Africa whereby if one is not dressed properly, the elderly would ask the person to return home to dress properly.

The wearing of a church uniform is part of the ritual healing process because it is not only about buying and wearing it but should be also sanctified by the pastor's prayers. I used to see members of the church buying uniforms and presenting them to the pastors to pray and bless them. Generally, the church uniform in the Zion Christian Church is considered holy apparel; hence, women are not allowed to touch the male uniform and the other way around. I observed that when it happened that a woman touched the male uniform by mistake, they would call the pastor to pray so it could be sanctified. This also explains why members of the Zion Christian Church would not wear their uniform to an ordinary event or wear it in public but rather only when going to church. This is because the church uniforms are considered holy apparel such that even when going shopping I observed that women would be in normal clothes and wear uniforms for church purposes alone. It speaks to the sacredness of the wearing of church uniform; it is supposed to be treated with deep respect and dignity. Even when storing the church uniform at home in the closet or the wardrobe, it is supposed to remain sacred and not be treated like ordinary apparel. Traditional healers in traditional African religions have a way of dressing which should be differentiated with church uniform in the Zion Christian Church. After all, it is not only the African Independent Churches but also mainline Christian churches that embrace the wearing of church uniforms. Therefore, it is not entirely true that African Independent Churches like Zion Christian Church have integrated traditional African religions into the wearing of church uniforms. On church uniforms, Sundkler (1961:232) concurs that a sick may be instructed to put on a certain uniform by the prophet and failure might result in the severity of the illness. This does not in any way connect the wearing of church uniforms in the Zion Christian Church with traditional African medicine.

Growing up in the Zion Christian Church, I observed that only mature men and women would wear the green uniform because it was considered very sacred. This uniform is called *seaparo se seholo* in Northern Sotho, which is translated as the sacred uniform. It is meant to be worn by the elderly and respected members of the church and not by children. This means that even the children of the baptized members are not allowed to wear this kind of uniform as it is only reserved for those who are mature members of the church. Even among the mature members if one engages in unholy acts, you would not be allowed to wear this uniform. This explains the sacrality of the yellow uniform among the mature members of the church, the majority of which would be pastors, particularly among men. This does not mean that ordinary men are not allowed to wear the yellow uniform but would be distinguished from the pastors by their collars. I observed while a member of the church that pastors should wear a yellow braid on the collar, whereas ordinary men would wear a plain collar. The main point is that this type of uniform represents some form of dignity among the church members. Again, this signifies the importance of this type of uniform in the Zion Christian Church and the status that goes with the wearing of such a uniform. Moreover, it connects to the ritual healing process in the sense that only those who are considered holy and mature can wear such a uniform, or else sickness can come upon those who are not eligible. Furthermore, those wearing this type of uniform would also be required to sit in front of other congregants to demonstrate the power and authority of this uniform. Therefore, it should be reiterated that the green and yellow uniform is considered the most sacred uniform only to be worn by men and women of integrity and not young men or women, let alone the children of baptized members.

The khaki uniform worn by the male members of the Zion Christian Church serves as a protective measure in a similar way to the military uniform. In the church, the colour of this uniform signifies spiritual warfare against the spiritual forces causing sickness and disease. In addition to the khaki uniform, the male members of the church would wear a cap on their head bearing the star of the church right in front. A cap like this is worn by other members of the community, but something that makes the Zion Christian Church cap different is the star placed on the front of the cap. It must be reiterated that the male children of the baptized members as discussed above are allowed to wear the male choir uniform as they also partake in the *mokhukhu* services with their parents. It is thus common for the parent to bring his son along when attending the *mokhukhu* service. The women in the Zion Christian Church also have their choir, and they are also allowed to wear their khaki uniform. However, in distinguishing between the male and the female, the women would also wear a blue uniform. It is therefore common to see women in their blue uniform rather than the khaki uniform to ensure that they are distinct from the male choir which is limited to the khaki uniform. Nonetheless, the point made here is that the male choir uniform demonstrates the authority that these men have to engage in spiritual warfare in confrontation with the evil spirits. This is different from the garments worn by the traditional healers who seek to connect with the spirit world, particularly the ancestral spirits. Therefore, here again, we see some dissociations between the wearing of garments in the traditional African religions and the church uniform in the Zion Christian Church.

More than the uniformity, the wearing of church uniform in the Zion Christian Church has other deeper meanings and connections to the spirituality of the members. In the first place, the church uniform has a bearing on the spiritual protection against the evil forces that cause sickness and disease. Those who are wearing the church uniform feel protected against spells and misfortunes which are responsible within the framework of ritual healing for causing sickness and disease. Once in their church uniform, church members feel fortified and protected against the forces of darkness. Therefore, in the Zion Christian Church, the wearing of a church uniform is considered a place of safety against sickness and diseases. Secondly, the wearing of church uniform in the Zion Christian Church makes the member sacred or holy. Put differently, when wearing the church uniform, the member is encouraged to adhere to the fundamental teachings of the church and also to the laws and protocol of the church. Thirdly, the wearing of a church uniform is considered a healing ritual as the church member can wear the uniform to receive healing. Lastly, a member of the Zion Christian Church can feel more powerful or at a place of authority over sickness and disease by wearing a church uniform. As opposed to ordinary apparel, it does not only give the member dignity but also a sense of power and authority. Hence, the members of the Zion Christian Church would sacrifice anything for the purchase of the church uniform. Thus, it is more than ordinary apparel but a sacred and holy one. The church uniform in the Zion Christian Church, particularly the green and yellow, carries with it some form of authority and ranks the member higher than others; hence, wearing green and yellow affords one an opportunity to occupy the front rows during the church service. Therefore, the wearing of church uniform in the Zion Christian Church also affects the seating arrangement whereby those wearing the green and yellow would be seated in front of everyone else. Those who are not wearing the church uniform would be required to sit at the back which again points to the hierarchy of the wearing of church uniform. Most importantly, this speaks to the authority and power that comes with the wearing of a church uniform. This explains why those who are not wearing uniforms would feel a bit alienated from the church and not have a sense of belonging while attending the church service. This connects the wearing of church uniform with spiritual protection in the Zion Christian Church which should be differentiated from assimilation to the spiritual world in the wearing of garments amongst traditional healers in traditional African religions.

The sprinkling of water mixed with sand

Water in the Zion Christian Church is used on its own as what is referred to as holy water. However, water is also mixed with sand to pour on premises such as homes, businesses and farms to serve as protective measures in the Zion Christian Church (Mashabela 2023). The water that is mixed with the sand is not ordinary but would be collected from streams and rivers. Members who come from coastal areas such as KwaZulu-Natal, Cape Town and Gqeberha (Port Elizabeth) would be asked to bring water and sand from the sea. This kind of water is popularly known as *meetse a leshata*, which is directly translated as noisy water which also means living water. Thus, the water from the sea, the rivers or even the streams is considered living water. Similarly, the sand from the above-mentioned sources would be considered relevant to serve as protective measures for the members of the Zion Christian Church. Like the holy water discussed in the previous chapter, this kind of water that is mixed with the sand is blessed by the pastor through prayer. In addition, it is the pastor who is supposed to come upon invitation or instruction by the prophet to sprinkle or splash such water around the house, the business or even the farm of members of the church. Members cannot use the water that is mixed with sand on their own as they are not authorized to do so, and also the water would not be effective as it needs the blessing of the pastor. It is, therefore, quite common to see a pastor sprinkling or splashing the water that is mixed with sand around the houses of Zion Christian Church members to protect them against evil. We always have to remember that whatever is done in the Zion Christian Church is to confront the evil spirit in the same way Pentecostals do. The difference is that in the Zion Christian Church, certain rituals are used, but I contend that these rituals like the water with sand should be differentiated from the practices of the traditional African religions.

The water that is mixed with sand is used to protect the household against the forces of darkness. Lukhaimane (1980:59) explains that 'water with some sand added to it was used to sprinkle homes, businesses, and even crops to ward off witchcraft or misfortunes'. This kind of water is used to sprinkle around the house in the yard, on the doors and on the roof of the house. Although sand would not be used, in a similar gesture, water would be sprinkled around the car to protect it from accidents and other attacks. Growing up in the Zion Christian Church, I used to observe pastors sprinkling water on cars even when the engines were opened to release protection upon the vehicles. It is therefore common for members of the Zion Christian Church not only to take their cars to Zion City Moria to receive blessings but also to be sprinkled with water for protection while driving on the road. It is also common that during major gatherings such as the Easter conference, members of the church would take their cars to Moria to be prayed for and blessed by the bishop with the same aim of protecting them on the road. The followers of traditional African religions would take their new cars home and present them to their ancestors to receive protection while driving on the road (Mbiti 2015). Many believe that failure to do so might lead to an accident or the car being stolen. Thus, while both members of Zion Christian Church and followers of traditional African religions seek spiritual protection even for their cars, the difference once again lies in the source of that protection.

The only disadvantage is that the water that is mixed with sand seems to be damaging the corrugated iron, particularly when it is splashed on the roof of the house or any other premise as discussed above. I have observed the same in our house when my late father used to splash this kind of water around the house and on the roof. This would leave marks on the corrugated iron, and at the end, there would be holes in the roof where water could seep through during the rainy seasons. Besides, the water that is mixed with sand also leaves marks on the roof that make it look untidy. But many of the church members just like my late father would not take any precautionary measures to prevent this corrosion of the corrugated iron; their priority at that time would be the protection of their household. Therefore, the members of the Zion Christian do not care whether healing and protection practices are not friendly to use or put differently can end up compromising the very people and their premises as is the case with the corrosion of the corrugated iron. However, it can be reiterated that the main focus of the followers or adherents of the Zion Christian Church is spiritual protection against witchcraft. Adherents would not care whether the protection and healing practice was compromising their life or not. Generally, Africans are always willing to do anything for spiritual protection against sickness, disease, misfortune and other evil forces. But again this should not be grounds for linking traditional African medicine with the ritual healing process in the Zion Christian Church.

Church badge

Another protective and healing ritual in the Zion Christian Church is the badge which is part of the church uniform but has different functions from the latter. In this book, the church badge is discussed by taking an in-depth look at these functions. Although I did not own a badge as I was not a baptized member of the church, I used to see my father's and mother's badges. I observed that among the features of the badge is that the name of the church appears on the Silver Star. In addition, I observed that each badge has both the rectangular shape green cloth and the round black cloth. I also observed a very little blue cloth which is normally placed between the rectangular-shaped and round-shaped clothes. All these shapes are put together by a pin attached to the silver star to form a badge. The star in the Zion Christian Church is used like the one in the Bible in Matthew 2:10–11 to provide direction to the believers, 'When the wise men saw the star, they were filled with joy. They came to the house where the child was and saw him with his mother, Mary, and they bowed down and worshiped him.' This means that when members of the Zion Christian Church wear the badge with this star, they would be able to be pointed to the headquarters of the church, that is, Moria, Boyne (Boyne refers to the suburb where Moria is located) where they will be able to worship God. This also means that once a member has been baptized and received the badge, it would not be easy for the member to leave the church. Therefore, the badge becomes a connecting point between the church member and the church itself such that they would not easily deviate from the church laws. Therefore, even the church badge in the Zion Christian Church is not used in conjunction with the traditional African religion but in observance of the church laws.

The church badge in the Zion Christian Church was first introduced by the church founder, Engenas Lekganyane in 1928 mainly for the identification of the church members (Lukhaimane 1980:72). This means that as the church grew to greater numbers, the only thing by which they could be identified among the crowds was through the wearing of the badge. Hence, while it is not permissible to wear the church uniform in public, it is permissible to wear the church badge (Moripe 1996). This is because this symbol was used for church members to identify each other, particularly when in public spaces. Hence, the Zion Christian Church members would greet each other in public even if they did not know each other. It is much easier to spot a Zion Christian Church member through the badge which is normally worn in visible areas on the garments of the individual member. Equally, in other places such as the workplace, sporting events, or even community meetings, it would be easy to identify a member of the church because of the badge. This is possible because upon seeing the badge, they can identify with the person and greet them with the peace rhetoric in Northern Sotho *kgotso a ebe le lena* which means 'May the peace of God be with you.' This is important because the church has millions of adherents across the globe; so by wearing a badge, they can identify each other. Wouters (2014:125) points out that not only are they able to identify each other but also help each other in times of need. When one member is involved in an accident, for example, the person is more likely to receive help from fellow Zion Christian Church members because of the badge. This is consistent with the spirit of ubuntu as an African Indigenous Knowledge system whereby it is not common to pass a person on the street without greeting them. This is not common in the Western world where individuals only care for their wellbeing. In this way, the church badge becomes a token of peace, fellowship and unity amongst the members of the Zion Christian Church. This also signifies the disconnections with traditional African religions where symbols of peace and unity are not identifiable.

The badge is also a symbol of allegiance to the church, meaning that wearing a badge means that the member agrees to adhere to the fundamental teachings of the church (Lukhaimane 1980:73). Hence, when a member feels that they want to do something wrong, they would first take off the badge so that they do not defile badge. One cannot, for example, drink or smoke while wearing the badge of the church. I do remember that most members of the church will be conscious about the rules of the church when wearing their badges. They would be able to remember all the restrictions and the code of conduct in the church. This means that the church badge serves as caution and in a way moves the members of the church away from bad behaviour and helps them to adhere to the fundamental teachings of the church. These teachings eventually help members to live a healthy life. Therefore, when seeing someone wearing a badge, one would assume that they are trustworthy and live a holy life as per the requirements of the church. If one member is tempted in any way, they would first remove the badge and only then engage in actions such as smoking or drinking alcohol. Another example is women who when not going to church would not cover their heads; in this case, they too would not be allowed to wear the badge. Members of the church eventually become members in good standing because of the simple symbol of the badge. In this way, the badge serves as a disciplinary measure for members of the Zion Christian Church whereby they think twice each time they want to engage in wrong behaviour. This means the badge serves as a symbol of solidarity, faithfulness and allegiance to the church laws. Therefore, when wearing the badge, church members would remain faithful to the church regardless of where in the world they might be.

The badge serves as a unifying factor, as all members of the church would be wearing it during church services. It is the one symbol that makes members of the Zion Christian Church look the same throughout the world. The one aspect of the badge that distinguishes it from wearing the church uniform is that it can be worn in public and outside of church services. Therefore, it makes it possible for members of the church to remain united even when they are not in church. This makes the church badge in the Zion Christian Church one of the powerful instruments of the church. When someone sees another person wearing the badge, it is as if they have seen family. Thus, the badge becomes the symbol that enforces oneness and unity among the members of the church. Lukhaimane (1980:73) explains, 'Members rallied to one another on recognizing the badge irrespective of the ethnic group to which they belonged. They were brothers and sisters in Christ and the Zion Christian Church.' Therefore, the badge serves as a symbol of bringing members together regardless of their diversity. Generally, members of the Zion Christian Church are considered one big family rather than a different and fragmented family because of the star. It is the badge that is responsible for bringing them together as one. This is an important factor since South Africa is a diverse nation that at times can be polarized among racial and ethnic lines. The badge in the Zion Christian Church has therefore been instrumental in serving as a unifying factor between church members. This is something also related to the African philosophy of ubuntu, particularly its aspect of the sense of belonging in the African context.

As much as non-members are not allowed to wear the church uniform, I also observed that non-members are not allowed to wear the church badge. This also means that non-members as discussed above are not allowed to just pick up the badge and wear it without having been baptized in water. Another reason is that baptism serves as induction in the Zion Christian Church where all other healing practices are introduced to the new member. Hence, non-members who are not familiar with the instructions would not be permitted to wear the badge. Like many other healing practices, the pastors should first bless the badge before it is handed over to church members. Once blessed, the badge serves as a healing practice that can be used when members face sickness and disease. I observed members of the church who would place the badge where they feel the pain to provoke healing. This placed a demand of the badge whereby even non-members would attempt to use the badge for the sake of accessing healing. Thus, the badge is one of the powerful instruments attracting non-members to the church who use their faith to access healing through the same healing ritual. Different healing practices are used but what matters is the patient's faith, which activates the healing. But I must point out that even when these members and non-members use these healing rituals, they still have to believe that they can be healed. This is important, that is, the role of the belief system in the ritual healing process where symbols and objects are considered as secondary rather than primary in the healing process. Therefore, it is not necessarily the badge that heals but the power of God.

The badge, like the wearing of a church uniform, is an icon of spiritual power used for the protection of church members; it is not just a sign of uniformity among church members. It demonstrates that the church founders such as Engenas Lekganyane carry certain spiritual power, and they have released this power onto something tangible like the badge. Lukhaimane (1980:73) points out that the badge is not only a symbol of faithfulness and unity in the Zion Christian Church, but it also serves as a symbol of protection against criminal elements. It is for the same reason that members of the church would not be easily robbed or attacked by criminals because of the badge. This is part of the healing practice because during attacks by armed robbers, one can get injured.

So, the badge can be considered a healing practice as it protects members against any bodily harm. Hence, different pieces of cloth are used in the badge including the little blue cloth hidden from the public as it serves as a protective measure for members of the church. However, Lukhaimane (1980:73) points out that some members of the public including the robbers themselves would discover the advantages of the badge and secure it for their hidden agendas. This happened because some members of the public discovered that preference was given to members of the Zion Christian Church because of their badge. The badge thus became an in-demand item because people wanted to receive the same favours as members of the church. However, the Zion Christian Church remains very strict in limiting the wearing of the church badge only to church members and considers it unlawful to wear the badge without first adhering to the rules and regulations of the church.

The badge in the Zion Christian Church serves as a symbol of peace within the framework of ritual healing. In other words, the members of the Zion Christian Church do not consider themselves as people of violence but as people of peace. This is one of the important aspects of the spirituality of the Zion Christian Church – it is founded on the peace rhetoric. Most of the time the members of the church and even non-members would greet each other using the same peace rhetoric which demonstrated that they believe in peace. When growing up in my village, the neighbours who were non-members would greet my mother and father in the same rhetoric and my parents would respond by saying 'let it be so'. Therefore, the badge is one such symbol that enforces the peace talk rhetoric among the Zion Christian Church members, meaning, when one sees someone with a badge, one is compelled to greet them using the same rhetoric. In this way, sickness and disease will not dominate the lives of Zion Christian Church members as they pursue peace in their daily lives. The spirituality of peace or rather the peace rhetoric is one of the hallmarks of the Zion Christian Church which in a way also becomes the healing practice. In summary, the badge in the Zion Christian Church does not only represent adherence to the church rule. I have observed that it is not only used for the protection of the church members but also to propagate the message of peace for both members and non-members. Therefore, the badge is not an ordinary symbol but one that is taken seriously by church members, and which is kept away from non-members. Most importantly, the badge is a symbol of peace, unity and fellowship. These values are important in identifying the distinctions between ritual healing in the Zion Christian Church and traditional African medicine.

The photographs of the bishop

Another protective healing ritual in the Zion Christian Church is the photograph of the bishop which is popularly known as *senepe sa mookamedi* in Northern Sotho. Members of the Zion Christian Church can acquire photographs of the bishops at the administrative office in Moria or main offices such as in the City of Tshwane. It is believed in the Zion Christian Church that if a witch enters the house and sees the photograph of the bishop, the witch will run away and not inflict the family. Therefore, it is the propensity of church members in the Zion Christian Church to purchase these photographs. One family will have the three photographs of Engenas Lekganyane, Edward Lekganyane and Barnabas Lekganyane which would mean that their house is well fortified against the forces of witchcraft. I noticed that the members of the Zion Christian Church perceive having the photographs of the bishops as a great honour. Therefore, having the photograph in the house of the church member is like having the bishop himself present in the house. I have heard many people over the years saying that the photograph of the bishop has a presence more like a living human being and serves as a source of protection against evil attacks, particularly witchcraft. This attests to the power that the photograph of the bishop carries at least as per the perception of the members of the church. For those who are in business, they believe that the photograph of the bishop would help in bringing customers to the business, particularly for those running shops. In addition, they believe that the photograph of the bishop serves as protection around the premises of the business and assists with the profitability of the business. Thus, this photograph is important to businesspersons in the Zion Christian Church as they know that their businesses are safe when they are absent from the premises as long as the photograph of the bishop remains there.

In the traditional African religious context, most people would have photographs bearing the pictures of their loved ones for memory or even for commemoration. This unlike the use of photographs for spiritual fortification is more like ancestral worship. Thus, as much as the Zion Christian Church members put the photos of their bishops in their houses and businesses, this should not be translated as the worship of the bishop. However, the common practice by the followers of traditional African religions in putting pictures of their parents and grandparents on the walls might signify ancestral worship. The difference is that the bishop of the Zion Christian Church cannot be an ancestor of all the members of the church but only to the members of his family. Therefore, his photo in the houses of his members does not signify ancestral worship. Even in traditional African religions, portrayals displayed in houses can be part of ancestral worship only if they are not for mere decorative purposes or to serve as a memory of the departed but rather to associate them with one's beliefs. I must be clear here that I am not in any way concluding that having a picture of a loved one, whether living or dead, means one worships them. Hence, the photograph of the bishop should not be misinterpreted as ancestral worship. However, we cannot at the same time underestimate the fact that in traditional African religions, some believe that having the photograph of the dead family member somehow retains some level of connection and can open some spiritual doors for them. Therefore, even in photographs, disconnections exist between traditional African medicine and the ritual healing process in the Zion Christian Church.

Strips of white cloth

The wearing of the strings or strips of white cloth which is known as *motlamo* in Northern Sotho is done in the Zion Christian Church for the protection of members against witchcraft which is also one of the causes of disease. The root word of *motlamo* is *go tlama* which means to arm or fortify yourself. The wearing of strips is done to also dispel misfortunes in the life of the believer or the follower of the church. Daneel (2019:46) explains that

> sanctified strips of linen cloth, are worn by women around their abdomen to stimulate fertility. The prophetically prescribed number of knots in it is supposed to determine the sex of the unborn child. Worn by children immediately after birth, or by grown-ups around their necks, arms, and legs, these strips serve to protect the body against visiting spirits.

However, the strips of white cloth are not only worn by women, even men and children are given the same to bring protection over their lives. This strip of cloth is not supposed to be washed with any detergent or else it would lose its essence and power. The main purpose of this strip of cloth is for the protection of the person against the forces of witchcraft and sorcery. It is believed in the Zion Christian Church that when a member is wearing this strip of cloth around their waist, the witches will not be able to touch them at night. Therefore, by wearing a *motlamo*, the patient is well protected against any infiltration by witches during the night. A *motlamo* is not supposed to be visible to other people but must be covered by the skirt or trousers around the waist of the patient. However, a *motlamo* around the waist of a child might accidentally be revealed during play, so parents discourage children from wearing this sacred cloth. Thus, a *motlamo* remains a sacred piece of cloth that is not supposed to be seen by others.

Other Zionist churches in Africa do believe in the wearing of a strip of cloth around their waist for protection against all sorts of evil. However, the colours and the type of cloth used for the strip would differ from one church to another. Some would use a very thin strip of cloth which is black and brown for protection against evil forces. Wearing a strip of cloth around the waist is a common thing in traditional African medicine. But again the difference is the functions of these strips of cloth. In the Zion Christian Church, a strip of cloth is worn to prevent evil spirits from coming into the life of the patient. Therefore, the members of the Zion Christian Church have a propensity to fortify themselves against forces of witchcraft and sorcery. *Motlamo* is also used as part of the indigenous knowledge systems to protect patients against future evil attacks that may cause further disease. This happens also among many members of neo-Pentecostal churches; they would wear wristbands but not necessarily the strips on their waist. However, in traditional African medicine, these strips also serve to connect one with the ancestral spirits. Thus, the use of strips in the Zion Christian Church should be distinguished from the use of strips in traditional African medicine.

Blue piece of cloth

Members of the Zion Christian Church also wear a blue piece of cloth which is known as *khutane* in Northern Sotho. Although it is compulsory to place it between the black and the green cloth on the church badge, I have also observed that it is also common for members of the Zion Christian Church to use *khutane* with other clothes as well. It is, therefore, common among members of the Zion Christian Church to attach *khutane* to their clothes as a way of protecting them against witchcraft. Members of the church who are serving in government as police officials, nurses or soldiers would attach *khutane* to their uniform for protection in the workplace. However, this is not supposed to be visible to other people as the word *khutane* itself means something that is hidden. Lukhaimane (1980:60) explains, 'The function of the *khutane* was to protect the individuals from assaults and lightning.' Therefore, the members of the Zion Christian Church would wear the *khutane* in the hope that they would not face challenges in the workplace, business and other social spaces. This means that one of the important things to do upon purchasing new clothes is to ensure that *khutane* is used in the clothes in addition to praying over and blessing them. However, the *khutane* is not popular for use among children; its use is widespread among adults who have been baptized in water. Children are deemed protected as long as they have worn the *motlamo* as discussed in the preceding section. However, it must be emphasized that *khutane* in the Zion Christian Church is not used as a spiritual connection to the spirit world as is the case in traditional African medicine (Last & Chavunduka 1986). However, in the Zion Christian Church, *khutane* is only used as a symbol of protection against the very spirits in the spiritual realm. *Khutane* does not like traditional African medicine give the members of the church certain powers to be feared or idolized by the people but rather only protects them against harm.

Brown paper

In protecting members of the Zion Christian Church against non-members, they would also be given a brown paper. According to Anderson (2001: 113), the members of the church are given this kind of paper to carry with them each time they visit non-members so that they are protected against any harm. If, for example, they are given food by non-members, they would be required to set the brown paper alight to protect themselves. This helps members in preventing food poisoning, particularly when visiting unfamiliar people or attending ceremonies where food is offered to them. Anderson (2018) provides another function of the brown paper which is placing it 'in the grave with the corpse, especially when it is believed that the deceased may have been bewitched. The brown paper protects the dead person against sorcerers, who may want to resurrect the body and use it for their evil purposes.' But this should not be defined as part of ancestral worship which happens in the graveyard amongst followers of the traditional African medicine. Besides, in Africa, people would use any protective measure against thieves who would steal the coffins to resell them to other clients. This is not an ancestral practice but a protective measure.

It appears to me that this brown paper in the Zion Christian Church is used for protection rather than for worship. Asante and Mazama (2009) explain that the use of artefacts, paintings and even the spoken word are used as rituals for the protection of the corpse. This is done through the use of brown paper in the Zion Christian Church so that the corpse is not stolen as it would interfere with the connection between the dead and the living. Ephirim-Donkor (2015: 151) cf Ephirim-Donkor (2016:177) points out that within the framework of ritual healing, Africans are very much jealous and protective of their dead; therefore, they would apply protective rituals to guard the corpse against any harm. These practices I argue here that they should be differentiated from the worship of ancestors which is done at the graveyard by calling the names of the dead for protection and blessings.

Copper wires

The copper wires which are known as *Mathale* in Northern Sotho are also important protective symbols in the Zion Christian Church. Some members of the Zion Christian Church would also use these wires, particularly on the inside of the door with the same aim of protecting them against lightning and thunder. The copper wires are normally placed at the gate of the yard in the homes of church members. This, according to Lukhaimane (1980:60), is used to protect members of the church against any form of lightning and thunder. The protection against lightning is important, particularly for church members who are living in rondavels with thatch roofs. It is important to point out that when the Zion Christian Church was started in the first quarter of the twentieth century, most people were living in rondavels, particularly in rural areas like the Transvaal, Natal and the Eastern Cape. Therefore, the church's revelation of using copper wires became important not only as a healing and protective ritual but also scientifically. This science is implemented now in the twenty-first century whereby even modern apartments would use copper around thatched houses to prevent them from being struck by lightning. But it is important to point out that in the Zion Christian Church, the copper wires are not only used scientifically against lightning but are also used spiritually to protect households against the forces of darkness, particularly witchcraft. Therefore, even though this proves to be a working scientific usage in guarding against lightning, it is used more spiritually in the Zion Christian Church. Besides the concept of lightning in African cosmology is not only caused by bad weather but also the evil spirits which is known as *tladi* in Northern Sotho. So *tladi* is not ordinary lightning but the one used by a witch to strike a house. Normal lightning in Northern Sotho would be called *legadima*, hence the need for the use of sanctified copper wires in the Zion Christian Church.

Africans are used to the idea of protection against lightning and thunder. This is because lightning and thunder are regarded as terrifying acts and people would be fearful if lightning strikes their houses. As a general practice, many believe that when lightning strikes, everyone should be indoors to avoid being hit by the lightning. However, Auerbach (2011:61) points out that the challenges of lightning can happen even when indoors.

> Lighting injuries may occasionally occur indoors, particularly from contact injury or side flashes from plumbing fixtures, computers, hard-wired telephones or electronic game devices, and other appliances. With hard-wired phones persons may suffer acoustic damage, neurocognitive deficits, death, or other lightning-related problems, because the phone system in most houses is not grounded to the house's electrical system and so acts as a conduit for lighting either to come into the home or to exit from it.

Therefore, lightning seems to remain a challenge whether when one is indoors or outdoors. Hence, churches like the Zion Christian Church do not only apply scientific measures but also spiritual measures to prevent lightning and thunder from hitting their members. This practice is also common ritual healing practice as the practitioners seek to protect their adherents or patients against the same. In doing so, ritual healing is not only used to protect against lightning but also to heal those who have been struck by lightning. However, this too cannot be linked to traditional African medicine but rather to indigenous knowledge of how Africans protect themselves against thunder and lightning.

Sticks

The male members of the Zion Christian Church are given sticks *dipatla* not necessarily to fight others but to serve as protection against any eventuality. I have observed that the sticks in this church can also serve as a protective practice against the powers of witchcraft. People who have struggled against the powers of witchcraft would receive help after joining the church (Anderson 2018:116). The lead singer of the male choir (*mokhukhu*) would carry these to serve as a protective measure during their dancing and praying. In addition, the church members would travel with these when moving from one city to the other. Therefore, it is also important to make a distinction between the long stick and the small stick which are both used during the dancing of the male choir. Nonetheless, the holy sticks are part of the ritual healing process in the Zion Christian Church. According to Anderson (2018:162), the sticks can be placed on the patient for them to receive healing. They can also be used to point in the direction of the pain in the body of the patient when praying for healing. Therefore, in the Zion Christian Church, when an individual is suffering from the spells of witchcraft, they would use sticks against the sources of witchcraft (Frey & Wood 2000). Moreover, it is important to point out that protection against witchcraft is an important thing in the Zion Christian Church as witchcraft is regarded as the cause of disease and sickness. These sticks are called by Sundkler (1961:229) 'holy sticks' that can heal the sick. Therefore, it is surprising that Sundkler (1961) would make connections between healing in the African Independent Churches and traditional healing since traditional healers do not use holy sticks.

Whip

The last protective symbol discussed in this chapter is the use of the long whip which is known as *Sefepi* in Northern Sotho. This whip is normally used with the stick that is held by the male members of the Zion Christian Church. They use it during dancing to dispel any forms of witchcraft and to protect members of the church. Wouters (2014:233) explains that the use of the whip is another healing and protective ritual in the Zion Christian Church which is used to dispel all kinds of diseases. When the whip is used during the *mokhukhu* performances, it is done so that they can dispel the power of *tokoloshe*. Hence, the *mokhukhu* performances happen during the night most of the time. The whip will also be used to protect houses, businesses and cars. Upon the purchase of a new house or car, the church member would call the pastor to pray and use the whip for protection. In addition, the pastors use the whips at the houses (old or new) of church members to fortify them against the powers of *tokoloshes*. In African mythology, a *tokoloshe* is believed to be a spirit that can be used by witches and sorcerers to invoke curses and to cause disease among the members of a certain family (Sibam-Twalo & Ally 2022). *Tokoloshe* is seen as a spirit that can torment human beings such that at the command of the witch, it can cause misfortune and other evil things to happen to an individual. Most Africans according to the study conducted by Sibam-Twalo and Ally (2022) in the Eastern Cape of South Africa believe in the existence of the tokoloshe not just as imagination but as the spirit that causes evil things among people. In the same study, Sibam-Twalo and Ally (2022:109) described the tokoloshe as having invisible powers which even though it is not seen are attested to by the misfortunes people experience. In dealing with the challenges of the tokoloshe and other evil forces in the spirit realm, Anderson (2018:121) explains that a whip is one of the protective and healing practices that the Zion Christian Church uses to deal with the problem of the *tokoloshe* among its members. Reeder (2012) says this whip is called a witch-whip, and it is used for casting out the evil spirits invoked by witches. It is believed that when the whip is used against the ground or even on the walls, it chases the *tokoloshe* away from a house or the people living in the house. Therefore, it is correct to point out here that the Zion Christian Church is dealing with the challenges of *tokoloshes* among the African people. In addition, when driving or walking around, especially during the night, the pastor of the Zion Christian Church is expected to carry a whip so that they can use it against possible attacks by criminals. Again, there is a connection between the protective rituals and the cause of sickness within the framework of the ritual healing process.

Conclusion

This chapter discussed the protective practices in the Zion Christian Church to find their connections with the ritual healing process. The chapter found that the members and followers of this church would use many of these practices as protective measures against disease, which implies that they are part of the ritual healing process. Church uniform (*seaparo*) is not only worn for the sake of looking good to other church members but also serves as a protective measure against attacks of sickness and disease. Members of the Zion Christian Church have a propensity to sprinkle water that is mixed with sand to protect their homes. The wearing of the badge is not only done for church members to identify each other when in public, but it also serves to protect church members against criminals, particularly in urban areas. Another protective healing ritual in the Zion Christian Church is the photo bearing the picture of the bishop which is popularly known as *senepe sa mookamedi* in Northern Sotho. The chapter also found that in the Zion Christian Church, the strings and strips are worn as armour against witchcraft. These strips and strings are worn together with the blue pieces of cloth to protect church members. The members of the Zion Christian Church also use what is known as the brown paper to protect them against non-members, particularly during visits. The use of copper wires at the gate of one's house is done to bring protection against witchcraft and sorcery. The male members of the Zion Christian Church use sticks to protect them against any eventuality or mishap while on the road. The church's male members, particularly during their *mokhukhu* (male choir) sessions, would carry the whip known as *sefepi* in Northern Sotho, which they use for protection. The study found that all these protective practices are used to fight against sickness and disease which has implications for the ritual healing process. In other words, once armed against any attack of disease, members of the Zion Christian Church would be able to live a healthy life. This chapter was also important in the disconnections between protective rituals in the Zion Christian Church and the use of some of the protective measures in traditional African medicine.

5

Therapeutic worship in the Zion Christian Church

Introduction

This chapter is an exploration of therapeutic worship in the Zion Christian Church. It seeks to demonstrate using ritual healing theory that the liturgical practices in the Zion Church are aimed at fulfilling therapeutic purposes rather than just observing liturgical orders. Therefore, this chapter seeks to illustrate that worship (including sermons) through the use of ritual healing theory is done to heal patients in the church. The different forms of songs of Zion including the singing of hymns are discussed here together with these ceremonies to understand their connection with healing practices. Praise and worship form an integral part of the liturgy in the Zion Christian Church and part of the various major ceremonies in the church. The Zion Christian Church believes in different gatherings which are also used to pray for the sick so that they may receive healing. Therapeutic worship is also experienced in other ceremonies such as *mpoho* (a night prayer that includes dancing and singing throughout the night). The chapter discusses the male choir (also known as *mokhukhu*) and the practices of the female choir whose worship practices have a healing effect. Other music groups in the Zion Christian Church include the *nkedi* group and the brass band which are both discussed in the context of ritual healing. Lastly, sermons that are offered in the branches of the church, particularly during Sunday services, bring healing to the lives of the patients. Moreover, the sermons ministered by Bishop Lekganyane are also expected to bring about healing to the people of God in this church. These aspects of the liturgy of the Zion Christian Church which are discussed here as part of the therapeutic practices in the context of the ritual healing process are distinguished from forms of music and ceremonies in traditional African religions.

Worship as a therapy

In the Zion Christian Church and other African Independent Churches, worship should be understood as part of the liturgy of the church. But unlike in the mainline Christianity in Africa, worship in this church goes beyond fulfilling a liturgical order to become a therapeutic exercise. In other words, when engaged in worship, particularly the singing of songs and prayer during the church service, the aim is not to entertain the audience but rather to heal the patients. Therefore, worship in the Zion Christian Church has ritual healing elements as opposed to ordinary singing in the church. It differs a great deal from the worship in mainline missionary churches where much singing is comprised of reading from the hymn book. In Africa, the majority of people expect to experience lively worship in the church as part of an African's love for music and dancing. Therefore, some would join the Zion Christian Church owing to its spontaneous worship. But I would add that it is not only about its spontaneity but also its therapeutic elements. I argued elsewhere (Kgatle 2019a:1) that the adherents of this church do not sing for the sake of liturgy but rather refer to a song as having healing elements such as invoking the healing power of the Holy Spirit. My late father used to say, 'It's not a song but a prayer.' He would say this each time he led the congregation into singing. Therefore, other song leaders in the Zion Christian Church would ensure that they sing songs that would intentionally be aimed at healing those who are facing challenges. Since music dominates the worship service in this church, it makes the whole spiritual service centred around the ritual healing process. Therefore, here we can see the difference between the Western forms of liturgy and the African forms.

Worship as therapy does not mean that singing will heal all kinds of diseases suffered by the patients in the Zion Christian Church. However, the ritual healing process is accompanied by the singing of different worship songs in the liturgy of the Zion Christian Church. Although therapeutic worship is not aimed at a particular patient suffering a particular sickness, the point made here is that it would generally be a healing moment during therapeutic worship. Nonetheless, we cannot underestimate the power of therapeutic worship in its ability to directly translate into physical, emotional or even psychological healing. It is also important to point out that worship becomes even more effective where the cause of the sickness is spiritual, as was the case with Saul as described in 1 Samuel 16.14–23. Saul was sick as a result of the evil spirit coming into his life after God's Spirit left him. Saul was advised to call a worshipper who would play a lyre and worship for Saul to get well. 1 Samuel 16.23 states, 'Whenever God's spirit came to Saul, David took the lyre and strummed a tune. Saul got relief from his terror and felt better, and the evil spirit left him.' In this case, it is evidenced that worship becomes more effective in exorcising the evil spirit that caused the sickness. Worship resulted in healing Saul. Ritual healing is instrumental in tracing the cause of sickness and providing healing. In this case, worship is pivotal in dealing with the root cause of not being well and providing healing.

Worship through singing, although it cannot heal terminal illnesses and diseases, can provide holistic therapy to the person, thus providing healing to the body, soul and mind. In other words, worship according to Kidwell (2014:129) can treat the spiritual needs of the person which may affect their physical well-being. Lazar (2005:195) describes worship as an activity that produces a positive experience which alone is important for the ritual healing process to take place. So even if patients at times are not directly healed by worship, the latter can release a positive energy that might end up motivating sick people to rise from their sick beds. It is for this reason that in the Zion Christian Church, worship is taken seriously as part of the ritual healing process. In support of Lazar's (2005:195) idea of a positive experience, I have added:

> Worship has a profound impact on the well-being of adherents. It makes people very happy to use their gifts to improve the happiness of others and ultimately their own. Worship in a church setting offers church members an opportunity to express themselves in the presence of God, which in a way brings them happiness. (Kgatle 2019a:5)

Therefore, worship can inspire and motivate the patient to such an extent that this can lead to therapy as it is the practice in the Zion Christian Church. In this way, the ritual healing process happens without the involvement of bishops such as Engenas Lekganyane or others because the source becomes the therapeutic worship in singing and dancing during spiritual services. It is for the same reason that the bishops would ensure that they are ushered in by music groups before taking the podium for preaching, for example. This will be discussed in the following sections.

Worship in the African Independent Churches is not done through talent alone but rather with the agency of the Holy Spirit. It is this aspect of worship in these churches that brings healing to the souls of those who are sick. Meaning, that churches such as the Zion Christian Church believe that singing connects them with the power of God that can release healing energy to the sick. This means that these churches are not engaged in ordinary singing and dancing but inspired by the presence of the Holy Spirit. It is expected during therapeutic worship that the Holy Spirit would touch the worshippers as they sing and pray along with the music groups. Therefore when singing, the worshippers provoke the power of the Holy Spirit as it has the power to seal with sickness and diseases. This is what separates singing by reading a hymn book and singing as led by the Holy Spirit, the latter contains the ritual healing elements through the power of the Holy Spirit. In this way, worship becomes a catalyst that plays a role of invoking the power of the Holy Spirit which is important for the healing of people or patients. Worship serves as a medium through which the patient can have an encounter with the Healer or the Divine power for the release of healing. The call on the power of the Holy Spirit is done in the same quest of making the church relevant to African people. In other words, the church believes that the Holy Spirit can meet the needs of the sick and the disillusioned. The allegiance to the work of the Holy Spirit in worship among African Independent Churches should be separated from the music and ceremonies done to invoke the ancestral spirits within traditional African religions. This is the difference that scholars such as Sundkler (1961), Hanekom (1975) and Mokgobi (2014) fail to make in their comparison of African Independent Churches and traditional African Religions. Hanekom (1975), for example, has failed to distinguish between the Holy Spirit in the Zion Christian Church and spirits in the traditional African religious worldview. He has mistaken the Zion Christian Church as being in continuity with the ancestral worship and in discontinuity with the Christian Holy Spirit. While scholars such as Mokgobi (2014:5) refer to prophets being possessed by the Holy Spirit, in the Christian language, we rather speak of being filled with the Holy Spirit than being possessed with the same.

Besides being directed to the patients in uplifting their spirits when facing sickness and diseases, worship also becomes therapeutic to the patient's family members. Should the patient lose their life, worship becomes therapeutic to the family in bereavement. Therefore, worship in the form of singing becomes important during funerals in comforting the members of the bereaved family. Different music groups would be called upon during these ceremonies so that they provide healing during bereavement. In the Zion Christian Church, this is very much central to the growth of the church as the members readily receive support from the church when faced with the loss of loved ones. The point made here is that such support comes through therapeutic worship when healing songs are sung.

Therapeutic songs of Zion

The worship in the Zion Christian Church is also studied by exploring the songs of Zion. Every member of the Zion Christian Church is expected to know various songs that are sung at the church. These would be comprised of the hymns that are popular in South Africa such as *A le mpotsang tsepo yaka, ke tlare ke Jesu*, meaning 'When you ask about my hope, I would say it is Jesus'. However, there are also songs that were uniquely compiled in the Zion Christian Church, such as *Mpoho* or even *Jesus o rile ke a tla bjalo ka lehodu la boshego*, meaning 'Jesus said he would come as a thief in the night'. I observed that most of the songs sung by the members are considered to be ministering hope and healing to the congregants, particularly those who are sick. In addition, most of these songs will be sung in the African languages so that they are sung with both the spirit and the understanding. As Paul pointed out to the Corinthians in 1 Corinthians 14:15, 'So what shall I do? I will pray with my spirit, but I will also pray with my understanding; I will sing with my spirit, but I will also sing with my understanding.' Although it is correct to say that all the songs are compiled into the songs of Zion, it must be noted that not all songs are original songs of Zion or were originally compiled by the church. As I highlighted above some of the songs were taken from the hymn books in the mainline churches such as the Lutheran Church and so forth. Nonetheless, every member of the Zion Christian Church is expected to sing along when the song is started by the congregants. However, even with songs that have been taken from mainline Christianity, I observed that they are sung differently as the Zion Christian Church combines the indigenous elements with the Christian message in the singing of the same songs. Although there are lead singers in the male and female choirs, it is permissible during the Sunday service for songs to come from the congregants. These include the male and female congregants of the Zion Christian Church who feel led by the Spirit to lead in a song. In most classical Pentecostal churches, the lead singer is assigned by the worship team leader, and it is therefore not so common for people to sing from the floor. Again, the Zion Christian Church can be seen as a game-changer when it comes to the music. But most importantly, these songs are sung as being led by the Holy Spirit which is different from the music and ceremonies in traditional African religions.

The Zion Christian Church is known for singing hymns, particularly in Northern Sotho which is again another element of indigenization. The singing of the hymns is expected to bring healing to the patients. I need to reiterate that the singing and dancing in the Zion Christian Church is done to provoke the power of the Holy Spirit so that the patients can be filled with the same power and be healed. It is therefore expected that during the singing of the hymns, the healing power of the Holy Spirit would descend on the patient. Therefore, the singing of hymns in the Zion Christian Church is part of a ritual healing process to invoke healing to the patients. It is common, therefore, for the sick person to be placed in the middle of a worship group in the Zion Christian Church so that the healing power of God can touch the person (Anderson 1991:101; 2000:165). This should be distinguished from traditional African medicine where normally a person possessed with demons would be in the circle while others sing to appease the ancestral spirits. Nonetheless, the hymns in the Zion Christian Church are part of the ritual healing process because they contain messages of hope, love and faith so that the patient when listening to them is encouraged to believe in God for healing. This connects with the Christian faith in the singing of hymns about the use of faith for healing but disconnects with the traditional African medicine in how the patients are healed through singing.

There are popular musicians in the Zion Christian Church who are known for singing the songs of Zion. Moripe (1996:56) explains that in the Zion Christian Church, 'artistic talents are utilized to the full, in the form of art, music and oral communication'. These include among others the late Oleseng Shuping, who became a force to be reconned with in the Zion Christian Church. Oleseng also started a group called 'The Atteridgeville Happy Boys' which also compiled and recorded songs of the Zion Christian Church. What made Oleseng so popular is that he was one of the first musicians to sing with musical instruments such as an organ and guitar whereas many before him just used vocals. Other musicians who became as popular as Oleseng are Stocks Nkosana and the late Mojeremane. The trio, that is, Oleseng, Nkosana and Mojeremane formed a group called 'The Rock' that also sang the songs of Zion. In addition to the trio, the other male artist who rose to fame for performing the Songs of Zion is Kenny Mankweng; the latter like Oleseng also used musical instruments. Other than these four, the male choir which will be discussed in detail below also recorded various songs that the members of the church can listen to. There are also female artists in the Zion Christian Church such as the group *makgarebe a bochabela*. Early on in her career, the popular musician Winnie Mashaba was also known as the singer of the Songs of Zion. However, she has lately distanced herself from the church and joined groups such as Songs of Praise which is known for singing popular and modern gospel songs. Nonetheless, the point made here is that when these artists sing, it is expected that healing will take place among the patients listening to the music. In addition, these artists listed above can also be considered Christian gospel song singers as they sing to communicate the Christian message more than popular religions in Africa. These artists do not sing only based on their talents but are also expected to sing as per the leadership and inspiration of the Holy Spirit. Hence, their songs are expected to heal the hearts and souls of the adherents of the Zion Christian Church. It is therefore correct to say that Zion Christian Church musicians are part of the ritual healing process in the church through therapeutic songs. And since many of them were baptized in the church, they understand the other healing practices that go with the singing of the songs of Zion. In the next section, this study explores the different important gatherings in the Zion Christian Church.

Therapeutic major gatherings

The church has different gatherings that are held throughout the year with the primary purpose of worship. The first important gathering (which is *kopano* in Northern Sotho) is during Easter. The second one is the gathering normally held during the first week of September at the church headquarters, Zion City Moria. However, it is the Easter gathering that is attended well. It has previously attracted leading politicians in South Africa, even during apartheid, particularly during the leadership of Edward Lekganyane (Anderson 1999). Political leaders such as PW Botha, as highlighted in Chapter 2, used to come to Moria, during the middle of the twentieth century. In the last quarter of the twentieth century, we saw leaders such as Nelson Mandela, Mngosuthu Buthelezi and De Klerk visiting Zion Christian Church in Moria. This was important then as these leaders wanted to not only worship at the church but also pray for peace in South Africa. In the twenty-first century specifically in 2012, we saw leaders such as Jacob Zuma and Julius Malema visiting the church, also for prayers and blessings. The Easter gathering is the largest and attracts thousands of attendees who come to worship God at the headquarters of the Zion Christian Church. In most of the Easter conferences, people would come from different countries in the region, and others would come from overseas in some conferences. Therefore, these conferences are always well attended, and at times, there is no space for both people and cars. This is an indication that the Easter conference is well attended and attracts millions of adherents of the church from different countries in southern Africa. This points to the popularity of the church and the leaders in the African continent. In 2014, the bishop welcomed visitors from all over the world:

> Whereas we have always acknowledged individual members of the ZCC from America, Canada, Oceanic, and Oriental countries, including of course [the] central African region and our branch in the United Kingdom, today it gives me great pleasure to acknowledge the presence of our representatives from Saudi Arabia in the Middle East. (Maahlamela 2017:130)

These major gatherings are important as the bishop himself, whether Engenas, Edward or Barnabas, would preach the sermon addressing the delegates in attendance (Morton 2018). It is also during conferences such as Easter and the September gathering that it is expected that the bishop would confer God's blessings on the adherents of the church. It is during these gatherings that members would try to come as close as possible to the bishop. The hope for the members of the Zion Christian Church in getting close is to directly receive the prayers and blessings that they would not receive when they are not physically present at Moria (Wouters 2014:84). Business people would take advantage of a gathering called *lekgotla la baipereki* which is directly translated as the 'gathering of the entrepreneurs'. This gathering is also important for the members of the Zion Christian Church who are business-orientated to come and receive blessings at the church headquarters. This is an opportunity for those who would have missed a meeting with the bishop during major gatherings in Easter to also receive the prayers at Zion City Moria. Thus, the church members need to have contact with their bishop during major worship gatherings. However, since the church has a large membership, others would come to other meetings or as instructed through prophecy visit the church headquarters. The majority of the members of the Zion Christian Church believe that by touching the ground of the headquarters, Zion City Moria, they would receive their healing. Therefore, not only is the worship itself therapeutic, but the ground of Moria is also considered therapeutic, particularly during main gatherings.

But other than the Easter and September conferences, the church members of the Zion Christian Church would gather on normal Sundays for fellowship and worship. Normally, the Sunday services are attended by the local members in local branches across southern Africa and the rest of the continent. However, as highlighted above, a church member can receive a prophecy to attend the Sunday service at the headquarters of the church which they would have to obey. It is therefore very common for Zion City, Moria to have visitors on Sundays as some would have received prophecies. I have observed that the Sunday service normally starts in the afternoon just after 13:00 and lasts approximately four hours, finishing around 17:00 depending on the program of the day. This is different from many classical Pentecostal churches and other mainline Christian churches that start their services in the morning around 10:00. Therefore, normally when these churches finish their worship service in the afternoon, the Zion Christian Church would start theirs, which in my view is another factor that makes the church different. This again points to the significance of the church as a game-changer in the religious landscape. Different pastors would present their sermons on the day, but other activities would take place such as prophecies and the performance of various instructions alongside the Sunday worship service. It is also important to point out that during the service patients would receive prayers for their healing, and some would testify of the healing power of God. Therefore, members of the Zion Christian Church attend the Sunday service not only for the sake of fulfilling a liturgical order but also for therapeutic purposes. Hence, some would take their healing practices as discussed in chapters 3 and 4 for the pastors to bless them during the Sunday service. This makes this service, together with other major gatherings in the Zion Christian Church, therapeutic and should be understood as part of the ritual healing process in the African Independent Churches. Moreover, these major gatherings should be discussed in the context of Christian gatherings as opposed to gatherings in traditional African religions.

Therapeutic *mpoho* ceremony

Mpoho is a ceremony of dancing and singing during the night to pray, normally conducted on Saturday night in the Zion Christian Church (Maahlamela 2017). *Mpoho* in simple terms is a night vigil where worship takes place throughout the night which is consistent with other evening spiritual events in the African worldview. Unlike the Easter conference which is held at the headquarters, *mpoho* would happen in the homes of ordinary members of the church. A prophet would instruct a specific member to conduct the ceremony of *mpoho* after which the members of the branch and the surrounding branches would be present to pray with their fellow members. *Mpoho* is a ceremony that needs the approval of headquarters and is not always prescribed for families but only when a certain family is facing difficulties that cannot be solved through normal prayers and instructions. *Mpoho* in the Zion Christian Church is also used for purification purposes but should be differentiated from the ceremony of *go tloša*

Setšhila sa lehu, which is also used to cleanse and purify a household that faced death within traditional African religion (Semenya & Letšosa 2011). Setšhila in traditional African medicine means that when one is faced with death, they become impure for a certain period which can be a few months depending on the tribe. In the Zion Christian Church, there is a belief that one becomes impure when faced with the loss of a loved one, going to the graveyard and so forth. However, prayers would be made during the *mpoho* ceremony which is different from the *go tloša Setšhila sa lehu*. The latter which happened in traditional African religions is where the members of the bereaved family are required to perform certain rituals including appeasing the dead some months after the death of their loved ones to cleanse and purify themselves. Although *Mpoho* is also prescribed in the Zion Christian Church to serve the same purposes of cleansing and purifying the church members who recently faced death in their families, it is done through prayer rather than appeasing the dead. In this case, *mpoho* is done through a Christian practice of prayer and worship during the night. Therefore, there are disconnections between ceremonies such as *go tloša Setšhila sa lehu* in traditional African religions and *mpoho* as a ritual healing process in the Zion Christian Church.

Something else that disconnects *mpoho* from traditional African religious ceremonies such as *go tloša Setšhila sa lehu* is the slaughtering of a cow that is normally dedicated to ancestors (Mankga 2013). These sacrifices where a cow is slaughtered are part of other cleansing ceremonies in the traditional African religions. Chitakure (2017:64) points out that cows slaughtered at ceremonies or even during funerals should not be taken like normal food as the cows are more about cleansing and to a certain extent part of ancestral worship. In some sections of society, such a cow would have undergone certain rituals before being slaughtered and offered to the people. Similarly, in ceremonies such as *go tloša Setšhila sa lehu*, there is also the slaughtering of cows or any other animal as part of the cleansing and purification ceremonies in traditional African religions. Therefore, *mpoho* should be differentiated from these ceremonies where even if food is served, it is not necessarily for ancestral worship. Besides, if one family, for example, cannot afford to offer food for delegates, they would opt for the second option of *mpoho* called *Phiri e Chaba moso*, which directly translates as 'a hyena is afraid of the dawn'. This concept is used to refer to the idea that members who cannot afford the provision of food during *mpoho* can opt for releasing their delegates early in the morning. Because if people are not released early, they would expect food in the morning. This again proves that in the Zion Christian Church, the purpose is not the slaughtering of cows which are dedicated to idols but rather the prayer for the members of the family who lost their loved ones.

It is also important to point out that during the *mpoho* ceremony, the attendees are expected to chant about the *mpoho* song repeatedly. Hence, scholars such as Wouters (2014) and Maahlamela (2017) described *mpoho* as a song rather than a ceremony. They also discuss *mpoho* as a music group rather than a ceremony. However, for this book, it is important to discuss *mpoho* as a ceremony to unpack the disconnections with traditional African medicine. When I was still in the Zion Christian Church, we would sing *mpoho* non-stop accompanied by dancing, particularly by men. Here also it can be discovered that *mpoho* is not just a song but part of spiritual warfare confronting evil spirits. It is through this kind of chant that the *mpoho* becomes an exercise beyond normal singing and becomes some form of prayer. While singing it, the lead singer would emphasize that *a se kosha ke thapelo*, meaning *mpoho* is more than a song: it is a prayer chant. *Mpoho* is more rhythmic and poetic connecting to African forms of poetry. Maahlamela (2017:137) calls it an endless song; hence, in the Zion Christian Church, it can be sung throughout the night. Songs like these should be differentiated from songs sung in different ceremonies within the framework of traditional African religions. In ceremonies such as *malopo*, there is also some form of chanting as part of calling the ancestral spirits when initiating traditional healers. Sundkler (1961:22) explains that 'the repeated performance of singing and dancing to a tune is required to please and materialize the spirit in whose honour the song is composed'. However, Sundkler's failure to identify that, *mpoho* is different lies in the fact that it is sung not to appease the ancestral spirits but to confront the evil spirits responsible for witchcraft and misfortune.

It is corrected to point out that *mpoho* both as a ceremony and as a chant is done as part of the ritual healing process. This statement is made because it is expected that people would receive their healing and deliverance during the singing of the *mpoho* song. But it is also correct that *mpoho* both as a ceremony and as a chant is part of the spiritual battle; hence, as a ceremony, it is conducted during the night. During the chanting of *mpoho*, the chanters would repeat the phrase *ka dinaka ya tlaba* referring to the horns of the cow saying that they can pierce through the enemy. It appears to me having attended the *mpoho* ceremony many times in my upbringing that *mpoho* is a ceremony designed for a spiritual warfare through which the adversary in the form of evil spirits and witchcraft are confronted. So by referring to the piercing horns of the cow, it is implied that during the *mpoho* ceremony, the enemy would be pierced and defeated. Maahlamela (2017:136) concurs by saying that '*mpoho* is also known as *kwadi ya marumo* (an ode of spears). *Kwadi ya marumo* denotes a battle song, yet [it is] spiritual.' This means that by singing *mpoho* and engaging in a *mpoho* ceremony, the Zion Christian Church members are engaged in a spiritual battle against the evil forces. This is consistent with the songs of battles sung by psalmists like David such as Psalm 24 meant not only for cleansing but also to fight spiritual battles. They are not, I must reiterate, associated with ceremonies in the traditional African religions. In the next section, I discuss the male choir as part of therapeutic worship.

The therapeutic male choir (*mokhukhu*)

An important group during worship in the Zion Christian Church is the male choir which is known as *mokhukhu*. The historical developments of the name *mokhukhu* for the male choir happened under the leadership of Edward Lekganyane when he seceded with his brother Joseph Lekganyane after the death of Engenas Lekganyane (Anderson 2000:173). The word *Mokhukhu* refers to the Northern Sotho word for the shack which is very popular in the townships in South Africa. This is because the followers of Edward did not like the followers of Joseph, hence the demand for the burning of their shacks. It is common when engaging in protests like this against the other factions that people would do it while singing and dancing; this is how *mokhukhu* became popular. Therefore, the etymology of the word *mokhukhu* about the male choir developed as a quest to burn the shacks of the supporters of Joseph who was the opponent of Edward at that time. This means then that the *mokhukhu* was formed more as a protest group singing and dancing in support of their leader, Edward Lekganyane. However, over the years, it outgrew its protest character to become a formidable spiritual music group in the Zion Christian Church. Nevertheless, the character of engaging in a spiritual battle remained in the *mokhukhu* music group. But the battle changed from people's shacks to a spiritual battle of fighting the evil spirits with their singing and dancing. *Mokhukhu* must be understood as a group that was formed to engage in factional and political battles in the Zion Christian Church but later became a spiritual music group engaged in spiritual battles.

The *mokhukhu* performances are done during their ceremony, which normally happens on Wednesday and Friday nights. The male members of this group are known as the 'Bafana ba *mokhukhu*' which loosely translates to 'the choir of the boys or men'. In addition, the male choir is also expected to perform during the *mpoho* ceremony discussed above, particularly in the early morning of the day after the ceremony. Moreover, the *mokhukhu* performs during the major gatherings of the church such as the Easter and September gatherings. It is not common for the *mokhukhu* to perform during the usual Sunday service as they are normally expected to sit and listen to the sermon. The wearing of the white boots popularly known as *manyanyata* is an important part of the uniform as members are expected to stamp their feet on the ground several times during their performances. Hence, younger men who still have a great deal of energy join the *mokhukhu* performance as it is expected of them to sing and stamp their feet during these performances. The performances are not held in the church but around the church. I have observed that the *mokhukhu* group would have their own small corner where they would be singing and dancing. Therefore, singing, dancing and stamping of feet dominate the *mokhukhu* performance. I have also observed that the dancing is not done haphazardly but rather in a very organized way where all members do the same dance moves at the same time. This is possible because there will be a lead singer directing the rest of the group. The performances of the *mokhukhu* group are consistent with the ritual healing process as part of the liturgy of the Zion Christian Church. This means that their performances are aimed at healing those who are sick whether present or absent at the performances. But these performances should be separated from the singing and dancing in the traditional African religions.

The lead singer is the one who is expected to be at the centre and lead the choir into different songs and also instruct them as to when to stamp their feet on the ground three times. However, other young men with the capability to sing in the church would also be allowed to take up songs and lead the *mokhukhu* in the singing of different songs. Hence, the *mokhukhu* performances can last for about two to three hours during which different lead singers would lead the song as instructed by a senior *mokhukhu* member (normally the one holding the stick). During the dance, the *mokhukhu* performers have constant contact with the ground sometimes with some of the performers touching the soil with their tongues. Some performers would also take up the soil in their hands while performing. It is important to point out that the *mokhukhu* performance does not happen on pavement but rather directly on the ground to make contact with the soil. When performing at the home of the church members during the *mpoho* ceremony, the *mokhukhu* performers would insist that they be given a special area where they can easily dance and stamp their feet; hence, pavement would not be an option. Contact with soil for spiritual purposes is an important aspect of taking over territories. But this should be separated from the contact with soil in traditional African religions as part of ancestral worship (Olupona

2014). Therefore, African Independent Churches make contact with the soil to demonstrate authority in the spiritual realm and not as part of ancestral worship. It is also believed that when people want to control one's destiny within traditional African religions, they would take up the soil where there was contact with the same person. However, these are not the intentions of the *mokhukhu* in the Zion Christian Church. The purpose of *mokhukhu* performers when making contact with the soil is to place their authority on the ground of the family member where the ceremony such as *mpoho* is taking place. This means that after the singing and the dancing by the *mokhukhu* group, it would not be possible for the evil spirits to torment the family again as the performers have taken over as spiritual authorities in the family.

The therapeutic female choir

The female choir in addition to the male choir is a popular group that also sings as part of the ritual healing process. The female choir normally gathers on Saturday afternoons and sings during the *mpoho* ceremony. They also sometimes sing during the main gatherings in Zion City, Moria. Unlike the *mokhukhu,* I have observed that the members of the female choir can have different moves while singing together. Nonetheless, a senior member of the choir would be the one to lead them in terms of arranging the lead singers and the seating arrangement. The female choir just like the male choir is expected to sing the songs of Zion that invoke the Holy Spirit to bring healing to the patients. Rafapa (2018:17) explains, 'The Zion Christian Church female choirs elicit the same fusion of symbolism as their Mokhukhu male counterpart.' Therefore, the female choir in the Zion Christian Church does not sing for entertainment but as part of the ritual healing process to invoke the power of healing to the patients. Most of the time, it is the lead singers of the female choir who would then lead the church into singing during the Sunday service as the members of the male choir hardly sings during Sunday service. The female choir is also important during the funerals of Zion Christian Church members as they are expected to lead the mourners into singing throughout the funeral service. Just like the *mokhukhu* who have young boys as part of the group, young girls are also part of the female choir and are expected to dress in the church uniform during their choir practice, the Sunday service and major gatherings at the Zion City, Moria. However, uniforms are not compulsory for all the groups during the *mpoho* ceremony, especially the night session of the ceremony. The members would rather dress in uniform in the morning when they are expected to sing before the congregants.

The female choir is also active during the Wednesday women-only service which is more like the *mokhukhu* male-only service on Fridays. The pastor would be assigned to attend this women-only service in case someone needed prayers or for those who came with certain rituals to be prayed for and blessed by the pastor. Although women are allowed to give sermons in church, they cannot become pastors. Hence, there is a presence of the male pastor during their services. The presence of the male pastor is also important for the cleansing of all women before they enter the sanctuary as it is considered a holy place. I have observed that this would be done in a way that as women come in to start singing in the choir, there would be a minister who would be ready to sprinkle water on them. In addition, I have also observed that the minister would sprinkle water in the area where they will be singing and dancing so that it remains a sacred and holy place. Therefore, the women's choir plays an important role as a therapeutic music group in the Zion Christian Church. The presence of the male pastor should not be seen as interference or lack of confidence in women's leadership but rather as part of the purification codes that exist in the church. Most importantly is that the female choir more like the male choir should be understood as part of the spiritual warfare against the evil spirits in the spiritual realm. These music groups I reiterate should be differentiated from the ancestral worship performed during various ceremonies in traditional African religions.

The therapeutic *nkedi*

Another important music group in the Zion Christian Church is *nkedi*. The *nkedi* group is characterized by Scottish-looking attire and performs in smaller groups as opposed to the larger groups such as the male and female choir. The fieldwork conducted by Wouters (2014) in Marabastad demonstrates that the *nkedi* group in that branch was comprised of the male members of the Zion Christian Church, particularly the younger men. However, in my observation, the Ga-Mamaila branch of the Zion Christian Church included women in the *nkedi* group. Therefore, *nkedi* can be considered a music group in the Zion Christian Church for both men and women. The uniform of the women *nkedi* group is similar to the Bapedi traditional attire. Therefore, it appears that the *nkedi* leans more towards a cultural music group than a religious music group as in the case of male and female choirs. This is illustrated by how the attire of *nkedi* resembles that of the *kiba* cultural group. The *nkedi* attire also includes rattles made out of dried seeds strapped around their ankles which is similar to the attire of *kiba*. The main function of these rattles is that they create a certain traditional rhythm during the singing and dancing. Like other music groups in the Zion Christian Church, the *nkedi* group is also expected to sing songs that would bring healing to the ill. However, the main point made here is that *nkedi* is aligned to a cultural group *kiba* more than the religious groups within the traditional African religions. This is an important point within the framework of ritual healing process whereby some rituals are aligned with culture rather than religion. Therefore, linking African Independent Churches with the traditional African religions through therapeutic music groups like *nkedi* is very unfortunate.

The *nkedi* group is not only connected to *kiba* but also to *dinaka*. Maahlamela (2017:155) describes *nkedi* as 'a *dinaka* (horns) ensemble free from reed pipes and drums. Drumbeat, here, is replaced with heavy staccato stomps of military boots wrapped with seedpod leg-rattles; reed pipes melody replaced with a spiritual and more encrypted sound-poetry.' But *dinaka* in the Northern Sotho culture and tradition is more than horns; it is a cultural group that plays horns as their main activity. Maahlamela (2017:155) compares the culture of *dinaka* with that of *nkedi* in the Zion Christian Church because of the rhythmic resemblances. However, there are also connections between *dinaka* and *nkedi* in the context of ritual healing process, meaning the two not only connect culturally but also in terms of healing. Maahlamela (2017:157) continues to say that '*nkedi* sound poetry is rooted in ambiguous and incoherent yet dynamically merged poetic phonaesthetics, embodying abundance of spiritual experience and evocation. This call-and-respond anomatopoiac words distinctly emulate reed-pipes melody of *dinaka*.' This in a way connects the *nkedi* musical group in the Zion Christian Church with ritual healing process particularly the *dinaka* group as argued by Maahlamela (2017). When both *dinaka* and *nkedi* play their instruments or sing and dance, the primary purpose is to invoke the Divine powers. In the *nkedi* group, the power of the Divine is invoked to bring healing to the sick. Hence, *nkedi* like other music groups in the Zion Christian Church can be considered a therapeutic group. In addition, the *nkedi* group more than other music groups in the Zion Christian Church connects more deeply with the ritual healing process. Again we see a connection between the music group in the Zion Christian with the cultural group among the Northern Sothos. However, scholars such as Sundkler (1961), Hanekom (1975) and Mokgobi (2014) have mistakenly interpreted these links with traditional African religions.

The therapeutic brass band

The other music group in the Zion Christian Church is the brass band that is mainly used to usher in the bishop, particularly during important visits and gatherings at the church premises (Müller 2016). Lukhaimane (1980:53) explains, 'As a way of greeting and praying for the people Engenas would lead his brass band and march in front with his walking stick. He used to put on a Scottish kilt when he marched. During such occasions, people would climb in trees and on top of vehicles to be able to see Engenas.' Anderson (1999:297) explains that the climax during the Zion Christian Church gatherings is the entrance of the bishop with his band. Everyone would be astounded as they watched the grand entrance of the bishop. Since most of the gatherings are attended by politicians as discussed previously, Anderson (1999:297) continues to say that not even the politicians can steal the euphoria of the bishop with his brass band. The brass band plays an important role in attracting many people to the church. It is also important to point out that the members of the Zion Christian Church and adherents are interested in the brass band and the possibility of seeing the bishop during the main events or conferences of the church. This is one of the motivating factors for the members of the church to visit the headquarters, that is, to see the bishop ushered in by the brass band.

The brass band is also part of the ritual healing process in the Zion Christian Church. In the first place, the brass band would play the songs that are already familiar in the Zion Christian Church so that even though there are no vocals, the audience can easily follow the song. The compilation of the songs played by the brass band mainly comes from the songs of Zion. In the second instance, there are testimonies of people who were healed while listening to the brass band playing and when it ushered in the bishop, particularly during the leadership of Engenas Lekganyane. I have observed that the brass band is considered as one of the music groups carrying special powers for the healing of the patients. So rather than calling the brass band to come and perform for the sick in their home, prophets would instruct patients to go and observe the brass band to receive their healing. In my view, this is one of the reasons why some patients would be asked to go and live in Moria for their healing. It is because, unlike many other music groups in the church, the brass band is not available in local branches. Therefore, it is correct to point out that the brass band has a healing effect on the patients; hence, the bishop is accompanied by this group most of the time. These musical groups, particularly the brass band, should not be perceived as measures of entertainment in the church but as measures of healing in the framework of the ritual healing process. The last section discusses the bishop's sermons as part of the ritual healing process. Music and ceremonies are used here to call people to the Christian faith; this should not be associated with traditional African medicine.

The therapeutic sermons

The sermons of the bishop particularly those of Engenas would appeal to the audience as he preached in Northern Sotho, and multiple interpreters would interpret the sermon into different languages repeating after Lekganyane. Given the presentation of the sermons in the African language and the African style, the sermons appealed to many of his adherents (Mashabela 2017). This is the strength of the African Independent Churches and partly other Pentecostal churches who present their sermons in the local languages to be relevant in the local context. Depending on the local languages in a specific branch of the church, a sermon by local pastors can be interpreted into different languages. For example, in branches such as Pretoria and Johannesburg, the Northern Sotho sermons preached by the bishop would be interpreted into Zulu. However, in the Northern Transvaal, which is now Limpopo, the sermons preached by the bishop would be interpreted in Xitsonga and Venda. This is done to ensure that the sermons reach as many people as possible. Therefore, there has always been a quest at the Zion Christian Church to make the sermons of the bishop accessible to the local people which includes translating the sermons into their local languages. Other than the language used in the sermons, the same would be distributed through the church's magazine called *The Messenger* where the members of the church would have an opportunity to read the sermons. This would benefit even those who have not been at the gathering or a conference in a specific year.

At the early inception of the church, the Zion Christian Church was not that grounded on the Bible in the sermon presentation as opposed to the mainline churches. Lukhaimane (1980:103) explains that during the early stages of the church, the pastors and church ministers who served under Engenas because of high levels of illiteracy at that time could not read the Bible. Therefore, most of them would rely on the experiences of Divine healing and the performance of other miracles that they have experienced during the ministration of Engenas Lekganyane and would apply these with the local congregants. Lukhaimane (1980:103) explains further that even Engenas Lekganyane would not preach from the Bible but rather talk about the power of God to heal their people. In the end, their sermons become testimonies of the healing and miracles that take place during the services. This is the case in the Zion Christian Church where sermons are dominated by healing testimonies rather than preaching the Word. The advantage is that the same sermons would have a very strong therapeutic element where those who are sick would be encouraged to also receive their healing through the testimonies of others. Thus, sermon presentation in the Zion Christian Church is relevant to the African audience as opposed to the sermons in many Western missionary churches. No engagement of the Bible should not be seen as a deviation from the Bible as is the case in traditional African religions but as something that was caused by illiteracy in the early inceptions of the Zion Christian Church. This does not necessitate the labelling of sermons in African Independent Churches such as Zion Christian Church as 'clerical exegesis', as Sundkler (1961:192) has done.

The sermons by the bishops in the Zion Christian Church are also dedicated to addressing the political matters in the country, particularly when the politicians are present (Anderson 1999:294). This allows the presiding bishop to address the important issues facing the nation. Therefore, in the past bishops such as Engenas, Edward and Barnabas have used their sermons fruitfully to deal with matters of peace and stability in South Africa (Anderson 1999:294). This is also the strength of the church because they are known for advocating for peace and harmony through their spirituality. The sermons in the Zion Christian Church were also dedicated to teaching the new converts the rules and regulations of the church. Although the new converts would receive similar teachings during the baptism ritual, this was not enough. Therefore, the local pastors and to a certain extent the women who were allowed to teach on Wednesday used this time to teach the church members about the rules of the church. These rules as it is going to be explained in Chapter 7 form part of the ritual healing process because the observance of the same would make it possible for members not to fall sick. Therefore, the sermon presentation in the Zion Christian Church does not only form part of the ritual healing process as part of worship but also forms part of the taboos and restrictions in the church. Most importantly, sermon presentation is a Christian practice rather than a practice in traditional African religions.

Conclusion

This chapter discussed worship as part of the liturgy of the Zion Christian Church. The study found that, unlike other mainline churches in an African context, worship is more than a liturgy as it fulfils the purpose of healing. This makes the Zion Christian Church a church relevant for discussion on music as a therapeutic tool in African Independent Churches. This was illustrated through a ritual healing theory whereby it was found that different major gatherings such as Easter are organized for the primary purpose of bringing healing to the lives of the patients in the Zion Christian Church. Apart from the major gatherings, there are also popular ceremonies such as *mpoho* ceremonies which are also organized so that the sick can receive healing. The choirs such as *mokhukhu* are organized to lead the male congregants in singing and worship that is meant to bring healing to the sick. Similarly, the female choir does not sing to fulfil liturgical orders but rather to heal the hearts, minds and bodies of sick people in the church. These male and female choirs are organized to sing during various ceremonies including during funerals to ensure that they comfort the bereaved families. The other important choirs that were discussed in this chapter include *nkedi* and the brass band which too are organized to sing to bring healing to the sick. The chapter also pointed to the sermons preached at the local branches of the church and the main sermon preached by the bishop during the Easter conference which is meant to bring healing to the congregants. These aspects of the liturgy of the Zion Christian Church were discussed in this chapter as part of the therapeutic practices in the context of the ritual healing process. The conclusion is that worship in the Zion Christian Church should be studied and understood beyond liturgy as it is carried out as a therapeutic exercise. The therapeutic elements of worship in the Zion Christian Church demonstrate that the church is more connected with Christian practices than the practices in traditional African religions.

6

Therapeutic prophecy in the Zion Christian Church

Introduction

This chapter explores the therapeutic prophecy in the Zion Christian Church. The chapter argues that the prophecies in this Church are aimed at dealing with the root cause of illness and diseases and prescribing the correct remedies. This practice is done by the well-trained prophets in the Zion Christian Church who are known as *mabone*. The chapter will discuss the aspect of prophecy in the Zion Christian Church that is known as one-on-one prophecy. In this Church, prophecy is given to an individual by calling them and addressing them privately rather than addressing them in public. The Zion Christian Church uses a diagnostic prophecy whereby the prophet reveals the various causative factors of the sickness and diseases of the believer. The prophet in this Church takes the role of a diagnostician to trace the causes of sickness and diseases. However, prophecy is not only the diagnosis but also the prediction of the future where the events that are supposed to happen in the future are told in the present. This aspect of the prophetic gift in the Zion Christian Church will be discussed by also reflecting on previous prophecies as predictions of the future by leaders such as Engenas Lekganyane. This chapter will also look at some of the prophecies that are aimed at addressing the problems of witchcraft and misfortune. Another important part of the discussion is that after having diagnosed the problem, the prophet will then give the prophetic instructions known as *ditaelo* for dealing with such a problem. The various practices of prophecy are identified and discussed here to look at the healing implications of prophecy in the Zion Christian Church. The aim is to discuss every prophetic practice in the Church to make distinctions between prophecy in the Zion Christian Church and divination in traditional African religions.

The Prophets (*mabone*) in the Zion Christian Church

It is important to point out that the leaders of the many African Independent Churches fulfill the role of prophet in addition to other roles such as healers. Put differently, the prophets who are mainly leaders of the African Independent Churches are also expected to be healers. The African Independent Churches compared to mainline Christianity are very particular in the use of the title "prophet". Cabrita (2018:164) explains "Increasingly, charismatic young figures came to style themselves as divinely appointed "prophets" rather than officials vetted by the religious establishment". The prophet could be anyone as long as they have received the training or special grace to function as a prophet. If the prophet is still young, they would be required to be under the tutelage of someone senior for better training in the ministry of prophecy. Therefore, in the Zion Christian Church, there are female prophets as well as male prophets as long as they receive training for the same. The main requirement is the infilling of the Holy Spirit, which enables the prophet to get revelations by the same Spirit. This dismisses the assertion made by Sundkler (1961) and later by Mokgobi (2014) that African Independent Churches mix the spirits in traditional African religions with the Christian Holy Spirit. Thus, in the first instance, the prophet takes the function of the healer in the church such as the Zion Christian Church as being led by the Holy Spirit. Therefore, the prophets would have rooms in their homes where they could treat or help patients (Daneel 2019:34). Prophets are known for their connection with the supernatural power to bring healing to the sick. Therefore, healing in the Zion Christian Church is not only achieved by using healing practices but also through the consultation of a prophet-healer. The members of the Church do not only go to a service for fellowship and to hear the Word but also with the main aim of consulting a prophet to find out the root cause of their problems. The prophet's function is slightly different from way to pastors, but they also bestow blessings on people. Hence, Bishop Engenas Lekganyane as a founder and leader functioned as a prophet to heal and bless the people of God. The argument is that the function of the prophets in the Zion Christian Church is aligned with the Christian faith.

Leaders such as Engenas Lekganyane are known for prophecy in addition to healing and the performance of other miracles. In one way or the other prophets such as Engenas do move in the prophetic ministry, hence the growth and expansion of their churches in Africa. Lukhaimane (1980:29) explains that "[i]n the Zion Christian Church Engenas was the Chief prophet and the personality around which every activity of the Church revolved". It is for the same reason that the members of the Zion Christian Church esteemed Engenas Lekganyane highly and every word he spoke was taken seriously and as a prophetic instruction. As I outlined in the previous chapter, members of the Zion Christian Church would receive the sermon given by the bishop as prophetic words, hence they would not ignore it. Ignoring the words spoken by a prophet is detrimental to bringing sickness and diseases. Subsequently, it is also believed that the leaders who came after Engenas are also gifted in the prophetic and their words would also be adhered to as the former would have passed the gift to the next generations. It is for these reasons that the bishops, as prophets of God, in the Zion Christian Church are considered to be carrying powers to convey the blessings of God on followers. Most Africans believe that God has given all the power to his prophets and therefore he has assigned the responsibility of conveying blessings to them. Therefore, the members of the Zion Christian Church would consider Engenas and other bishops as prophetic figures such as Moses and others. However, according to Anderson (1999:291), the practice of pneumatic gifts such as prophecy decreased during the leadership of Edward Lekganyane as was discussed in Chapter 2. It seems that Edward Lekganyane relied more on his leadership qualities than the pneumatic gifts as was the experience during the leadership of his father, Engenas Lekganyane. However, even with this transition, it does not mean the church is aligned with the practices of Traditional African religions.

In addition to the pastors and church ministers, the Zion Christian Church has prophets who are known as *mabone* in Northern Sotho. The only challenge is that scholars such as Sundkler (1961), Hanekom (1975), and Mokgoba (2014) have confused the role played by the prophet and that of a diviner. Because both trace the origin of sickness and disease to the spiritual realm. Consequently, the scholars above made the connections between prophecy in the African Independent churches and divination in the Traditional African religions. In the fieldwork conducted by Anderson (2003:110) it was found that "A person who was not baptised would become a diviner, and a person through baptism could convert the spirit of divination into the spirit of a prophet". This means that in traditional African religions, the practice of divination exists but would take different forms depending on the spirit that exists in the prophet. If the prophet is used by the Holy Spirit, they become prophets but if used by other spirits they become diviners. In the Zion Christian Church, *mabone* would refer to the Holy Spirit and not any other source like divination. Therefore *lebone* continues to function in the gift of prophecy as led by the Holy Spirit. Therefore, similar to the Zion Christian Church, other African independent churches operate under the direction of the Holy Spirit. Therefore, there should be a thin line drawn between the source behind prophecy in African Independent Churches and divination in Traditional African religions.

Hence, Anderson (1999:304) warns us that the fact that both the prophet and the diviner know the cause of sickness and diseases does not mean that their source is the same. I would add that there are also differences in the content of the prophecies being delivered as much as there are differences in the source. In this way, we should take cognizance of the different forms of the practice of prophecy particularly when it comes to the content of the prophecy. Hence, Anderson's other study (2018) makes us aware of the continuities of popular religions on one hand and the discontinuities on the other. But it is correct to say that the prophecies given in the Zion Christian Church aim at the healing of the patient through the different healing practices utilised by the church, thus connecting with the ritual healing process. Therefore, when the prophet gives a prophetic word in the ZCC, the patient has to learn more about the sickness to be healed. This is not the same with divination in the traditional African religions which can be used for other selfish ambitions including witchcraft. This does not mean that all divination in the African traditional religions is negative but there are differences with practices in the Zion Christian Church. Therefore, in the study of the prophecies in African Independent Churches, we should not only look at the source of these prophecies but also their content or purpose. One should be able to point to the ability of both prophecy and divination in tracing the root cause of sickness but also point to their differences in both the source and content of their prophecies. This is one of the distinctions that scholars such as Sundkler (1961), Hanekom (1975), and Mokgobi (2014) failed to make in their quest to understand the African Independent Churches. They were quick to draw the similarities by ignoring one of the fundamental differences.

It is important to point out that *mabone* are sometimes asked to volunteer at the Church's headquarters in Moria during which they would receive further training and impartation to prophesy in their local branches. This is a process where *mabone* are required to serve in different activities of the church as they acquire training in prophetic ministry. Daneel (2019:36) explains that "In the 'City of Zion' or the remote clinics of the prophets, prophecy is made on behalf of the sick. The permanent prophets who reside in Moriah are sometimes agriculturists helping in the cultivation of the land, advisors to the Church gatherings". *Mabone* would also help during the major conferences of the Church, particularly the Easter conference. Most of the time it would be mature people who serve as *mabone* in the headquarters of the Zion Christian Church, some young women could be seen practicing prophecy and serving as the prophets in the Zion Christian Church. Therefore, prophecy functions as a platform from where the younger generation could participate as opposed to say pastoring where only men were allowed to be pastors of the church. Growing up in the Zion Christian Church, I have observed young female prophets who would prophesy in the church. Therefore, the prophetic ministry is an opportunity for both men and women to exercise their gifts in the Zion Christian Church. Similarly, it is a very common thing nowadays to find young women participating in divination. Some of them even leave school to become initiates. The next sections will be dedicated to outlining the various roles of the prophet in the Zion Christian Church.

The Prophet and the Spirit

Before giving a prophecy to the patient, the prophet would demonstrate that they are under the Spirit. The prophetic ministry in the African Independent Churches depends on the Holy Spirit's work and power. Lukhaimane (1980:43) explains, "In the Zion Christian Church the distinction was made to refer to the Holy Spirit as Moya o Mokgethwa, not just Moya, which can simply mean air. In the Zion Christian Church, the Holy Spirit revealed its existence in the power to heal, to drive evil spirits from persons, and in Prophecy". It is very common to hear *mabone* in the Zion Christian Church saying "ke tlelwa ke Moya" which means that the spirit is coming or dwelling in them. Or some would say "ke tswerwe ke moya" to describe that they are under the influence of the Spirit. It is therefore the Spirit that is expected to give them the specific word to the patient. Anderson (2003:108) describes this process very well:

> The prophet would usually manifest some sign that the spirit has taken control; thus the prophets would snort, cry, whistle, pant, jerk, and contort their bodies in different ways. Some would bend over as they walked, wringing their hands behind their backs. Others would be completely silent and behave normally.

These kinds of bodily gestures during prayer do not happen haphazardly as per the leadership of the Holy Spirit through the prayer of the prophet. Some of the prophets as I observed in the local branch in Ga-mamaila would start to speak in other tongues chanting "maita" many times demonstrating that they are under the Spirit and about to speak the prophetic word. Anderson (1999:299) explains that the prophet must discern when the Spirit is moving so that they can lead the Church to such a prophetic moment. It is after these different bodily gestures as described by Anderson (1999) that the prophet would then begin to speak prophetically to the patient. But it must be pointed out that these gestures which happen a lot during divination do not mean that prophecy and divination are the same things. The diviner may display the same gestures as being led by spirits and the prophet as being led by the Holy Spirit. The main difference as discussed in the preceding section would be seen in the content but not necessarily the gestures.

In the African Independent Churches, the Holy Spirit is perceived as the Spirit that has the power to cast out evil spirits (Daneel 2019:14). The African Independent Churches such as Pentecostal churches believe in the existence of different spirits in the spirit realm. However, they differentiate between the Holy Spirit and other spirits by placing the former as having higher and divine power over other spirits. This means that the role of the Holy Spirit in the prophetic ministry is not only the revelation of sickness and diseases but also the confrontation of evil spirits that have caused these illnesses. Therefore, churches such as Zion Christian Church acknowledge the Holy Spirit as the one that gives power to the prophet to use against evil spirits. In this way, the prophet relying on the power of the Holy Spirit can address the problems of sickness and diseases particularly as being caused by the evil spirits in the spirit realm. In the intersections between prophecy and Spirit, the Holy Spirit becomes the one who leads the prophet in the revelation of the cause of sickness and disease. Therefore, the Holy Spirit is pivotal in acting against the evil spirits as the main causes of diseases. It is not only the prophet who is expected to have the Holy Spirit, the believers are also expected to have the same Spirit to overcome sickness and diseases. This demonstrates the role of the Holy Spirit in the ritual healing process particularly in the practice of prophecy. Thus, there is confrontation against the evil spirits in the African Independent Churches when it comes to prophecy. This is different from the African traditional religions where evil spirits are not confronted but appeased through different ceremonies. It is also important to point out that the diviner only depends upon the connection with ancestral spirits to be able to give out the revelation whereas the prophet depends on the power of the Holy Spirit.

The emphasis on the role of the Holy Spirit in the prophetic ministry in the Zion Christian Church is part of the emphasis on Spirit baptism during water baptism within the framework of the spirituality in African Independent Churches. Daneel (2019:45) explains that each time there is water baptism in the African Independent Churches, there is also an expectation that the power of the Holy Spirit would come upon the believers in the similar way it did during Pentecost in the Book of Acts. It is the same power of the Holy Spirit that makes it possible for the *mabone* to see things in the spirit that they will be able to reveal to the patient. Similarly, the Holy Spirit is responsible for dealing with all other powers and spirits such as those causing witchcraft and misfortune. In the struggle against the evil spirits, the Holy Spirit plays a central role in empowering the prophet on revelation and diagnosis of the same. It is therefore correct to point out that the prophetic ministry in the Zion Christian Church is more pneumatological. However, divination in African traditional religions is also pneumatological, but the difference is that in the Zion Christian Church, it is the Holy Spirit that takes charge whereas divination recognises other spirits. In Traditional African religions, even the spirit of the dead (ancestors) is believed to be influential and play an important role in the divination process. Some Africans believe that the ancestral spirit can come back to visit them and reveal certain things to them to avoid danger or even misfortune. Whereas in the Zion Christian Church, pneumatology relates to giving credence to the work of the Holy Spirit. In this context, we see a discontinuity with African Traditional religions when it comes to pneumatological influence in the context of the prophetic ministry process in the Zion Christian Church. These dynamics need to be taken seriously to understand the continuities and discontinuities in the African Independent Churches such as the Zion Christian Church (Anderson 2018). It calls for scholars such as Sundkler (1961), Hanekom (1975), and Mokgobi (2014) to reconsider their position on the links they make between African Independent Churches and traditional African religions.

One-on-one prophecy in the Zion Christian Church

In the Zion Christian Church, prophecy is not given in public, but one might call it a one-on-one prophecy. I have used these terms elsewhere in my works (Kgatle 2019, 2021, 2023) to describe the practice of prophecy by calling the recipient or patient into a private space to specifically prophesy to them. This is different from what may be called public prophecy which can happen when a prophet stands on the podium to give a prophecy to an individual or a group. When the prophecy is given to an individual privately, it becomes confidential and avoids embarrassment to the recipient or the patient in the case of the ritual healing process. Anderson (1999:308) explains that "[p]rophecy in Africa often becomes an extremely effective form of pastoral therapy and counsel, mostly practiced in private, a moral corrective and an indispensable facet of the Christian ministry'. The idea is that an individual would receive a specific revelation through the work of the Holy Spirit that directly affects their lives. Even in instances where many people visit the house of the prophet, they would go one by one to receive their prophecies whereby the patients would enter one by one when visiting a prophet. The family members might sometimes be allowed to enter the room but no stranger would be allowed. This is another way in which prophecy is not practiced in Western paradigms the way sermons are presented. In Western prophetic definitions, a pastor normally delivers prophecy as a public affirmation of the Word of God as read from the Bible or preached from the podium. But the African Independent Churches like the Zion Christian Church take it further than that to give the prophetic word relevantly to the recipient.

To perform a one-on-one prophecy the prophet would call the patient outside the sanctuary into a corner where he/she would share the prophetic word with them. In churches such as the new prophetic churches, this would happen in a private room or the prophet's office. However, since the Zion Christian Church does not have offices in local branches, the prophet would just pick a corner and prophesy privately where other people could not hear him or hear. Anderson (2003:108) describes this process very well:

> The people being singled out were pointed at by the prophet, and they then had to follow. Sometimes the prophet clapped hands together to get someone's attention and then pointed with the hands held together in a praying posture. The status or rank of the person being singled out made little difference; a young unmarried woman can command one of the church leaders to follow her to the prophetic enclosure for counsel, and he must follow.

Under normal circumstances, no one can say no when the prophet is pointing out at the people to receive the prophetic word. Most of the Church members of the Zion Christian Church would oblige and follow the prophet each time they are called on to receive the prophetic word. The audience would be understanding and would not seek to distance the prophetic moment wherein one of them is receiving the prophetic word from the Lord. Although generally, Africans would also want to obey the spiritual authority of the diviner, it is important to point out that this does not immediately make divination in traditional African religions and prophecy in Zion Christian Church one thing.

Other than the one-on-one prophecy we cannot underestimate the role of prophecy in encouraging the whole church to pray or fast or engage in spiritual warfare as part of the ritual healing process. It is therefore important to point out that while an individual cannot be called to the podium and expose their issues before the public, it is a common practice in the Zion Christian Church to call the whole church into prayer. The prophet is permitted to use the prophetic moment to address the Church as a religious group. I can recall moments when the prophet even prophesied during the music group performances such as *mokhukhu*. Similarly, the prophetic word can be issued during the female choir practice where female prophets prophesy to their fellow women during their fellowship. In this case, prophecy moves from just being a private practice to individuals to the group. Lukhaimane (1980:76) recalls an incident whereby "[a] prophet would kneel and start saying, Amen [many times] and say God of Engenas [many times] says you must pray for your difficulties ahead". Under this kind of prophetic unction, the people would know that the God of Engenas is with them. But a mention of the "God of Enegnas" should not be interpreted as the worship of Engenas but rather as remembering God according to generations the same way the children of Israel would be told to remember the God of Abraham, Isaac, and Jacob. In addition, the prophet can single out a group of people where they are addressed in little groups of four or five (Anderson 1999:300). This happens when a prophecy is directed not only to an individual but his friends or family. Therefore, it is common in the Zion Christian Church to see a group of people being called out to receive the prophetic word or specific instructions. Anderson (1999:300) recalls a moment when he was called out together with his fellow researchers to receive instructions about fetching water from the streams. The point made here is that in all the moments as shared by scholars such as Lukhaimane (1980) and Anderson (1999), the goal is not to embarrass an individual before others but to rather encourage the whole Church as part of the Indigenous healing practice. This is important as we seek to understand the role of prophecy in the ritual healing process among the African Independent Churches. We should be able to make the distinctions between one-on-one prophecy and the public prophecy given to the group as is the case in the Zion Christian Church. In addition, we should make distinctions between prophecy in African Independent Churches and divination in Traditional African religions.

Diagnostic prophecy

Diagnosis of sickness and diseases is part of the ritual healing process as practitioners both in modern medicine and faith healing desire to detect the root cause of the problem. While the diagnosis of sicknesses and diseases in modern medicine takes place using modern technology, the diagnosis process in African Independent Churches takes place through the discernment of the Holy Spirit. Although the diagnosis of the sickness and disease may differ from one African Independent Church to the other, it must be stated that this process forms part of the healing process in most if not all of these churches. Daneel (2019:12) explains that "[i]n these circles, a diagnosis which is based on the widely accepted African belief in the personal causation of all ailments and misfortunes - such personal forces being the neglected family spirits, malignant alien spirits, witches or sorcerers – is both understandable and acceptable". The prophet in the Zion Christian Church can diagnose the root cause of the sickness to provide the proper prescription. Daneel (2019) calls the diagnostic type of prophecy the most common practice in African Independent Churches. Therefore, the goal of the prophet is to diagnose the real cause of the problems or challenges including sickness and diseases. If a prophecy is given without getting into the details of the root cause of the problem, it is somehow doubted as the expectations involve the diagnosis of the problem. Rather than questioning the authenticity of the prophetic word, the members of the Zion Christian Church would rather question a prophecy for being undiagnostic. The expectation is that the prophet should be able to tell the root cause of the problem and be able to provide a solution to the same, hence, the demand for the diagnostic prophecy as part of the ritual healing process. However, it is important as discussed previously that the diviner also can trace the root cause of the problem, hence the need to discern the source behind such a diagnosis to separate Traditional African religions from the African Independent Churches.

The prophet as a diagnostician can reveal things that others may not be able to know at face value. Therefore, the prophet as a diagnostician is tasked with the revelations of the patient's deep secrets. This is why so many Africans are keen to consult a prophet because of similar reasons for knowing the deep secrets in the realm of the spirit. In a normal diagnosis process, a patient does not necessarily tell the prophet their suffering but would leave it to the prophet to diagnose it to demonstrate that they are gifted and able to tell things without any prior knowledge. Anderson (2003:109) explains that "[f]inding the cause of the suffering is very important in this context, and this type of prophetic diagnosis may not always be wrong. The diagnosis may produce a psychological catharsis that benefits the afflicted who have a real fear of witchcraft". Therefore, the patient should not worry about telling the prophet about their problem. It is the task of the prophet to find out the root cause of the problem. This is in a way done to prove the authenticity of the prophecy because the prophet would not have had a prior knowledge of the causative factors of the sick and diseases but only revealed to them by the power of the Holy Spirit. Therefore, when the patient can see that a prophet knows the root cause of their problems, they somehow believe in the prescription given to them. This is exactly what happens with modern medicine whereby the prescription of the doctor is trusted based on the accuracy of the diagnosis.

The practice of a diagnostic prophecy has made the African Independent Churches very popular on and outside the continent. Anderson in his other work (1999:309) pointed out that the diagnostic prophecy is the most popular and common form of prophecy that attracts people to churches such as the Zion Christian Church. People are not only interested in a particular prophecy but in getting the details about the root cause of their problem. While prophecy exists in other Christian traditions, the prophetic ministry in the Zion Christian Church is unique in being able to trace the root of the problem, hence its popularity. Therefore even if the solution is not yet found, a diagnostic prophecy becomes therapeutic in the sense that the patient at least knows the root cause of the problem even before the solution can be found. Although the patient is aware of their problems, they are very interested in how the prophet can reveal them without telling the same issues to the prophet. This works in the psyche of the patient to an extent that they also believe that the prophet is indeed used by the Holy Spirit. However, the fact that Africans hope that they will be able to know the root cause of their problem in diagnostic divination within the Traditional African religion does not make prophecy and divination the same (Gumede 1990). I must reiterate that we should be able to draw out the differences.

The differences between the diagnostic prophecies in the African traditional religions and the Zion Christian Church are well articulated by Daneel (2019:40):

> One can safely assume that the diagnosis of the prophet, if compared with the traditional divination, usually runs parallel to that of the [traditional healer]. The difference is to be found in the medium through whom the extraordinary knowledge is obtained. The [traditional healer] relies on divinatory slabs, and bones for his [or her] extra-perception, whereas the prophet invokes the Holy Spirit. Furthermore, the prophet tends to label all spirits as malignant, while the [traditional healer] makes a more careful distinction between ancestral spirits.

Therefore, diagnosis in the African Independent Churches happens by being sensitive to the work of the Holy Spirit whereas, in traditional divination, it happens through the use of various mediums. Moreover, the point made by Daneel (2019:40) is that while the diagnostic prophecy seems to be in confrontation with various spirits in prophecy, the diagnostic divination seems to rely on the same spirits as a source for their prophetic mandate. In the African Independent Churches such as the Zion Christian Church, diagnostic prophecy can be done by a prophet in the local congregation. It is therefore not only the prerogative of the Bishop or the Church founder such as Engenas Lekganyane, later Edward Lekganyane, or even the incumbent Barnabas Lekganyane. Nonetheless, regardless of who is responsible for the diagnostic prophecy, the point made here is that it is different from the diagnostic divination. The differences are clear in terms of the source from which both draw their prophecies as pointed out previously.

The differences are not only seen in terms of the source of the problem but also in the quest to help patients both in diagnostic prophecy and diagnostic divination. Daneel (2013:43) also points to some differences when it comes to how both practitioners (that is the prophet and diviner) differ in terms of bringing the solution to the diagnosed problem:

> Upon diagnosis of the illness, the remarkable similarity between the [traditional healer] and prophet activities cease. Both of them find the origin of the disease in the disturbed communal society. Both recognise the bedeviling effect of the powers unleashed in the inter-human relationships and the threatening support of the spirits. But they stave off these powers differently. While the [the traditional healer] seeks a solution that accedes to the conditions of the spirits, the prophetic therapy bases itself on a belief in the power of the Christian God, which surpasses all other powers.

The diagnostic divination is not so keen on finding the solution to the challenges that Africans face from a Christian God but rather in consultation with the deity in Traditional African religions. This brings us to a traditional African religious view of deity where it is not only belief in the supreme being as a source of life but also the existence of other gods. Similarly, within the framework of diagnostic divination, the solution does not only come from the supreme being but also through the help of other gods including the ancestors. Therefore, there are some differences between the African Independent Churches and the traditional African religions when it comes to the diagnostic prophecy as part of the Ritual healing process in the Zion Christian Church. They rely on different sources when it comes to the solution to the diagnosed problem.

Prophecy as a prediction of the future

Prophecy in the Zion Christian Church can predict the events in the coming future. This was one of the strengths of the founder and Bishop Engenas Lekganyane as he was able to predict the defeat of Germany by Britain. This made Lekganyane one of the great prophets in African Independent Churches (Lukhaimane 1980). Anderson (1999:288) concurs that the ability to predict the future made Lekganyane great and the Zion Christian Church very popular. Anderson (1999:288) continues to say that "[i]n 1917, he prophesied the defeat of Germany by Britain, and when this happened a year later his prestige as a prophet and 'man of God' grew. Engenas was primarily seen as a unique prophet with extraordinary gifts of revelation and healing". Other than this specific prediction of the future, Lekganyane was regarded by his members to speak things that would concern their future, hence they took everything he said very seriously (Lukhaimane 1980:80). This also solidified the existence of the Zion Christian Church in addition to other practices such as healing. So prophets such as Engenas Lekganyane were popular in their time because he was not only able to diagnose the problem and offer help to the patient but was also able to predict the events of the future. This included possible attacks on his patients and/or members of the Zion Christian Church. It remains the function of the prophet to protect the patients through prayer and other rituals against possible attacks from the spirit world. When possible attacks are revealed to the patients, they can find means to deal with them. For this reason, prophecy is popular in the African context and elsewhere in the world.

However, is not only that the prediction of the future involves good things happening to an individual or even a country as was the case with Britain. Sometimes, it is the prediction of the afflictions that would happen in the future. It is also important to obey the instructions of the prophet to avoid those afflictions happening to an individual or the Church. This means that prophecy does not always please the patient but also warns them about the bad things that might happen in their lives. It is the same in the Traditional African religions whereby a diviner can warn an individual or a family about impending afflictions. The diviners conduct divination through the help of the ancestor spirits and the throwing of bones. Again, the difference is that through the work of the Holy Spirit, the prophet in the Zion Christian Church can reveal the events of the future, but the diviner would rely on other powers in the spirit realm to predict future events. Prophets through the power of the Holy Spirit can deal with challenges of misfortune and other evils in the spiritual realm. This presents some form of discontinuity with the traditional African religions when it comes to the prediction of the future as part of the prophetic process. But the point made here is that both can tap into the future and warn their patients of the possible events that can happen in the future. Therefore, it remains the task of the prophet or a diviner to mediate possible attacks upon the patient, hence churches like the Zion Christian Church have attracted many in the African context as they seek to deal with life's challenges before they happen.

Prophecies against Witchcraft

The prophetic word in the Zion Christian Church can come as a revelation of the people who are engaged in witchcraft activities. This is also informed by the African spiritual worldview in the belief in witchcraft and sorcery. Mafico (1986:400) in Anderson (2003:121) explains that "[t]he majority of Christians in Africa affirm faith in God but still ardently believe in such superstitions as witches, witchcraft, sorcery, magic, and the like". This is also informed by the African spiritual worldview in the fear of witchcraft whereby many people in Africa fear witchcraft. Some Western scholars according to Daneel (2019:23) have been ignorant of the reality of witchcraft in the African context. Hence, the Western missionary churches have been unable to deal with the challenges of witchcraft or rather the diseases that occur in people as a result of witchcraft. Even pastors and theologians in Africa who have been trained in Westernised theological institutions have to a certain extent failed to address issues of witchcraft. Mbiti (1976:8) tells the story of an African theologian:

> [w]ho had been trained in Europe, where he attained a doctoral degree in theology. After nine and a half years of study, after getting his junior and senior degrees, he had to return home with the excess baggage which consisted of the Bible in the various languages he had learned, plus works by Bultmann, Barth, Bonhoeffer, etc. On arriving home, there was a big welcoming occasion of relatives, neighbors, old friends, dancers, musicians and many others. During the dancing and jubilation, and after he had related his experiences overseas, there was a sudden shriek. It was his older sister who had fallen to the ground. When the well-qualified theologian suggested that she be taken to hospital, he was told that the hospital was far. The theologian was then told that the woman was demon-possessed. When the African theologian tried to refer to

Bultmann's explanation in the New Testament, he got shocked that Bultmann had demythologised spirit possession.

This is just but one example of how many in Africa have ignored challenges around witchcraft which the African Independent Churches such as the Zion Christian Church have used to their advantage. The ignorance of witchcraft is what has to a certain extent caused much reliance on modern medicine when it comes to healing in Western missionary churches as opposed to the African Independent Churches.

To some certain extent, this is what has caused the proliferation of African Independent Churches since witchcraft problems in Africa cannot be solved by modern medicine. The confrontation of witchcraft in these churches becomes part of the ritual healing process particularly when witchcraft is perceived to be one of the causative factors of sickness and diseases. Therefore, the African Independent Churches such as Zion Christian Church become a hiding place or place of refuge in which the power of witchcraft can be overcome through prophecy and prayer. The patients are interested in knowing who is behind their predicament when it comes to the challenges they face. Mashabela (2017:5) explains that "[i]n an African context, witchcraft cannot be avoided about misfortune or illness, and the Zion Christian Church offers an alternate hope with an African solution to these agonies. Members claim to be protected from evil spells (witchcraft), which is not the case in African Pentecostal churches and mainline churches". Hence, the discourse on the ritual healing process in the African Independent Churches has always involved the solutions to the problems caused by witchcraft. People believe that by joining the Church the issues surrounding witchcraft would be defeated through prayer and prophecy. Therefore, it is one of the important roles of the prophet to diagnose the problems caused by witchcraft among members of the Zion Christian Church. This is not done to point fingers at persons who are perceived as witches but rather to confront the powers of witchcraft to bring healing to patients as part of the ritual healing process. Lukhaimane (1980:16) explains that the Church is a place that offers the members protection against witchcraft through prophecy. This protection against witchcraft, as it happens in African Independent Churches, should be distinguished from the incitement of fear among those who consult traditional healers in traditional African religions.

Generally, the problems that have to do with barrenness, miscarriages, or complicated births are most of the time associated with witchcraft in both traditional African religions and the African Independent Churches

(Daneel 2019:42). However, it is important to note that in traditional African medicine, some of these problems may be associate with the ancestral spirits, particularly the spirit of the paternal aunt. Daneel (2019:42) goes on to explain that:

> [t]hese spirits are visualised in the form of apparitions, which literally 'grab hold of the uterus' to prevent birth or complicate it. The [paternal aunt] has the right to perpetuate her name through the children of her brother's daughter if she dies without offspring. She possesses this right by the bride price paid for her, and which in turn would enable her brother to obtain his wife.

The spirit of the paternal aunt within traditional African medicine can also possess the living children to a certain extent who would then start practicing witchcraft. It is the same reason that in African cosmology and mythology, a paternal aunt is an important member of a family to be respected and honoured to prevent problems with the children. Both African Spiritual practices of prophecy and the African Independent Churches such as Zion Christian Church are knowledgeable and able to determine the root of the problem during the diagnosis of the problem particularly when it is related to witchcraft or ancestral spirits. The patient would be required to take specific instructions to deal with problems like these, that is, miscarriages, bareness, and complicated births. Although the African Independent Churches have male followers, they have been able to attract many women as most of them have problems such as those mentioned above.

Therefore, it is important to point out that the diagnostic and predictive styles of prophecy are more functional in the revelation of the causes of witchcraft and misfortune (Anderson 1999:300). The prophecies on witchcraft are sometimes problematic as they can have revelations for people who are engaged in witchcraft. In some instances, these could be members of the same family or relatives. In a way, when it is revealed that a family member or a relative is bewitching the patient, it causes acrimony between family members. This is worse as discussed by Daneel (2019:38) when such prophecies involve the in-laws as it becomes the root cause of the acrimonies between for example married women and their in-laws. This can also lead to acrimony between the married woman's parents and the in-laws. In addition, the prophecy on witchcraft can also cause societal conflicts whereby some members of a specific community would be burned due to a prophecy on witchcraft. Hence, revelations on who is a witch in a family or a community should be taken cautiously to avoid such conflicts. However, some prophets would discern this possible acrimony and rather speak of the spirit of witchcraft which requires many prayers to be overcome rather than point to the person of the witch. The same happens in the traditional African religions particularly the practices of the sangomas who also reveal the names of witches in dealing with the root cause of the problem. But these are not a ground for equating divination in traditional African religions with the prophetic word in the Zion Christian Church. There is some form of leniency when it comes to the revelations of the identities of witches in the Zion Christian Church as opposed to the African traditional religious practices of prophecies. The latter is important in dealing with the acrimonies that might arise when it comes to revealing the names of witches during the prophetic healing process.

Prophetic instructions

The practice of prophecy in the Zion Christian Church involves prophetic instructions which are known as *ditaelo*. *Ditaelo* are instructions given by the prophet in the Zion Christian which according to my observation are more like the prescriptions given by doctors. These instructions are given to the prophet through the power of the Holy Spirit which are then passed on to the patient by the prophet. These prescriptions are most of the time made of the healing and protective rituals that were discussed in chapters 3 and 4. Therefore, to recap the prescriptions would consist of the following: Blessed tea, holy water, pricking using a needle, salted water as a laxative measure, the enema for the cleansing and purification of children's bodies, stones for steaming, purchasing specific uniform, the photographs of the Bishop, strings and strips to wear around their waist, a strip of blue cloth, the brown paper to protect them against non-members, the sticks and whip among male members of the church. However, these would not be prescribed generally and at the same time. They would be prescribed as per the need of a particular problem to the patient and or member of the Zion Christian Church. Therefore, *ditaelo* play a much bigger role as part of the healing and protective rituals in the Zion Christian Church. In addition, some of the ceremonies such as *mpoho* as discussed in Chapter 5 can be prescribed to an individual and or family as part of the healing and protective rituals. Therefore *ditaelo* in the Zion Christian Church are very specific to the condition of the patient and also, and they are prescribed in the framework of the healing rituals in the church. The prophet cannot prescribe something outside of the main healing rituals that are already available in the church. Therefore, the prophet would still rely on the voice of the Holy Spirit to give the correct instructions and prescriptions.

Once the prophet knows the root cause of the problem they can give the correct prescription to help the one experiencing challenges. In a way by being able to find out the root cause of the problem, the prophet's instructions can be trusted by the patient. In the fieldwork conducted by Anderson (2003:113) it was found that "[a]lmost every church member interviewed stressed the importance of observing the *ditaelo* ('instructions') given to be safe. These *ditaelo* are individualised secret and personal rules that the member may not divulge to anyone else". This means that the patient is not expected to tell others about the instructions but rather to obey them. The instructions are a common practice whereby an individual is given specific instructions on what to do to overcome their predicament. However, this is not a common practice in classical Pentecostal Churches which only preach the word. There are no consequences or threats for not adhering to certain instructions given by the prophet. The Pentecostal Churches that come closer to the Zion Christian Church in emphasizing obeying instructions are new prophetic churches that also focus strongly on diagnostic and prescriptive types of prophecy. Once a member of the Zion Christian Church has received specific instructions to deal with the root cause of the problem, they will also be told to take these instructions to the pastors to receive prayers and blessings. In most cases, a patient is not supposed to use the *ditaeolo* alone with the blessing of the pastor or in the presence of the pastor. It is for similar reasons that *ditaelo* cannot be shared among the members of the Church even if they suffer from a similar sickness or disease. In this way, *mabone* and *baruti* (pastors) work together as practitioners in the Ritual healing process in the Zion Christian Church.

The obedience to the instructions given by the prophet is important to receive healing in the ritual healing process in the African Independent Churches. Anderson (2003:111) explains that the person might fail to receive their healing not because the healing power does not exist but because they have failed to obey the instructions of the prophet. This makes the prophetic instructions central to the healing of the patient. Therefore, whatever the prophet tells the patient to do to receive healing should be followed rigidly by the patient. In the Zion Christian Church, the patients would go out of their way in adherence to the instructions of the prophet even when this comes at a high cost. For example, a prophet might prescribe the purchase of expensive apparel as part of the ritual healing process. The patient even if they have not budgeted for the apparel would ensure that they purchase the uniform to receive their healing. Therefore, it is very rare for the members of the Zion Christian Church not to obey the instructions of the prophet as they are aware that failure to adhere to the instructions is to their detriment. In his other work, Anderson (1999:304) states that if for example a patient was given an instruction in which they may fight bareness, they may remain barren for as long as they disobeyed the instructions. Therefore, prophetic instructions in the Zion Christian Church are more important than the diagnosis itself. It is of no use if one knows the root of the problem if the patient is unable to address it by paying attention to the prophetic instructions. Similarly, if the prophet instructs the living water from the streams, it cannot be other water but the exact one prescribed by the prophet. It is also important to note that since the healing rituals also contain protective measures, the prophet is also tasked with prescribing not only the healing rituals but also measures that would protect the family and their surroundings.

Although I tried to separate prophecy as diagnosis and prophecy as prescription, it is important to point out that during the prophetic process, these two happen at the same time. When the prophet shows the patient the root cause, it becomes difficult for the patient to ignore the instruction. In addition, revealing the cause inflicts some fear on the patient so that they are not able to reject the instructions. Anderson (1999:308) explains that "[t]he Zion Christian Church prophet attempts to give a Christian response to the built-in fears and threats of African traditional cosmology, particularly in the healing sessions, when the nature and the cause of the disease are given at the same time". The patient would be happy to know the root cause of the problem and receive the prescription and therefore not worry when the prescription does not work as it at least gives them hope when they know the causes. The prophet's ritual healing process is a complex one comprised of both the diagnosis and the prescription. Therefore, it is correct to speak of the prophecy of diagnosis and prescription as one prophetic process. It is worse when such prophecies have something to do with the witchcraft the congregant would obey. Nonetheless, the argument is that even with instructions, divination would differ with the prescription sin the prophetic process among the African Independent Churches.

The prophetic instructions are part of the ritual healing process because the prophet prescribes specific healing rituals for the patient to be healed (Anderson 2003:111). However, it is not limited to prescribing healing rituals, but would also prescribe modern medicine to heal the patient and this would depend on what a specific patient is suffering from. This as different from the position of early Zionists who would rely much on prayer and faith for the healing of patients and discouraged modern medicine (Cabrita 2018:2). However, the position on biomedical remedies should not be seen negatively as demonstrating devotion and love for God by forsaking other things. Cabrita (2018: 140) states that:

> early Zionists spoke of their miraculous experiences of healing as evidence not only of the power of God over sickness and Satan, but as signs of "the wonderful love of Jesus for them." They phrased their quest for bodily healing not only as a desire for wellness, but also as an overpowering "hunger for God," characterized by a "melting heart." Embracing divine healing and renouncing medicine was cast as devotion toward a lover, a leap of faith into the embracing arms of God.

However, I would argue that the Zion Christian Church is accommodating to biomedical remedies as opposed to other African Independent Churches which only prescribe healing rituals and oppose biomedical treatment. Therefore, it must be explained that in African Independent Churches, a prophet functions more than a biomedical practitioner. However churches such as the Zion Christian Church are not necessarily opposed to biomedical treatment. However, it is the members who would insist on seeing a prophet to trace the spiritual cause of the problem. Hence, when some people are afflicted by physical pain such as a fractured leg, they would insist on visiting the prophet for similar reasons of finding out the unknown cause of the accident or incident that led to the fracture of the leg. However, in traditional African medicine problems such as fractured leg would always be associated with witchcraft instead of providing a biomedical solution. Therefore, once again we see some disconnections between divination in traditional African religions and prophecy in the African Independent Churches.

Conclusion

This chapter looked at one of the important aspects of the spirituality of the Zion Christian Church, namely prophecy. The chapter linked the practice of prophecy with the ritual healing process in the sense that prophecy is not only the word given to an individual but rather the measure used to trace the root cause of sickness and diseases among the members of the Church. The chapter looked at various trained prophets in the Church who work as prophets in local branches. One of the functions of the *mabone* in the Zion Christian Church is to call out the members of the Church and give them a prophetic word in secret as opposed to public prophecy. Another function of *mabone* is to trace the cause of the sickness or disease that the patient is experiencing to provide the relevant prescription. *Mabone* in the Zion Christian Church also knows the events of the future including the various battles or conflicts between countries. As discussed in the chapter, Engenas Lekganyane was able to predict the defeat of Germany by Britain. Therefore, Bishops such as Engenas Lekganyane do not only function as the leader of the church but also as the *lebone* of the church. The chapter also looked at the specific prophecies in the Zion Christian Church that address the issues of witchcraft and sorcery. The challenges would require specific instructions as opposed to ordinary sickness and diseases. This brings us to the last but not least important aspect of prophecy in the Zion Christian Church which is the instructions and prescriptions given to the patient to deal with the root cause of the problem. This phenomenon known as *ditaelo* is important in the church as it was discussed as a "do or die" process in the Church that members would seldom ignore for their good. The chapter aimed to demonstrate that all the prophetic practices in the Zion Christian Church are part of the ritual healing process of the Church. In addition, it demonstrates the disconnections between divination in Traditional African religions and prophecy in African Independent Churches. This changes how we study and understand the gift of prophecy in the African Independent Church. Prophecy in churches such as Zion Christian Church is done as per the leadership and instruction of the Holy Spirit whereas in traditional African religions, divination is done as per the connection with the ancestral and other spirits in the spiritual realm.

7

The social restrictions in the Zion Christian Church

Introduction

This chapter discusses the social restrictions, taboos and holiness in the Zion Christian Church that have therapeutic and protective implications in the life of the believer or members of this church. The church has many taboos that contribute to the well-being of the believers in the church. For this reason, the Zion Christian Church was the first to agree to the government measures of social distancing during the Covid-19 pandemic. One of the types of taboos or restrictions in the Zion Christian Church is on food, particularly the prohibition of eating pork and animals that died of illness. Additionally, the women in this church are expected to dress respectfully for their well-being. This chapter also discusses the fact that smoking and drinking are discouraged, particularly among the church ministers, as a measure not only of social restrictions but also of holiness. Other restrictions exist in the church concerning death, how funerals should be conducted and how members should behave during such ceremonies. There are also restrictions concerning the ceremonies regarding the unveiling of the tombstones of the members of the church. The members of the church whose children have attended initiation schools are not supposed to go to church for a certain number of weeks. The headquarters of the Zion Christian Church itself is considered a sacred place with many restrictions, particularly for visitors who have to obtain permission before visiting the site. These social restrictions and taboos are discussed as part of the ritual healing process. In other words, each social restriction and taboo is looked at in terms of how it contributes to the healing or health of the members of the Zion Christian Church. In addition, each social restriction is discussed to dissociate the same with traditional African medicine.

The Zion Christian Church and taboos

Moripe (1998:9) defines taboo as 'a basic element of the religious experience and attitude of man/woman. It originates from an instinctive fear of or awe towards the mysterious 'other' world and its powers by which men/women feel surrounded.' Taboos exist primarily for monitoring behaviour in African life. This means that when Africans observe the taboo in their life, they can live longer. Although some taboos are common among many tribes in Africa, taboos might be specific to a clan or tribe or, in this context, a particular religious group. Some sicknesses and diseases are believed to have been caused by the non-observance of a taboo by an individual or a family. Life would be in an imbalance once there is a disrespect of the restriction placed upon a family or community which might result in serious repercussions. This makes the taboos and social restrictions part of the ritual healing process. Moreover, the observance of a taboo can lead to a healthy lifestyle, as prevention is better than cure. This means that when the members of African Independent Churches such as the Zion Christian Church observe the taboo, they can prevent sicknesses and diseases, which is better than seeking healing when one is sick. Therefore, as we discussed in the last chapter, in tracing the disease through the diagnostic prophecy, the prophet can identify the non-observance of a taboo as a causative factor of the sickness or disease. Furthermore, in tracing the cause of misfortune, the prophet can conclude that non-observance of the taboo is the cause. Therefore, they would try to observe the taboo to prevent misfortune. Diviners are also able to link sickness with non-observance of a taboo, but as discussed in the previous chapter, the difference with the prophet would be the source that provides such a revelation.

The non-observance leads to impurity, or, put differently, Africans observe taboos to avoid being impure. Therefore, Africans would seek the knowledge of what makes one impure so that they can avoid impurity. Many in Africa are aware that non-observance of a taboo may lead to consequences such as long illness. Hence, they would avoid the taboos, including getting close to a person who is considered to be impure. In the Old Testament, the person who had leprosy would be certified unclean to avoid being in contact with other people because they would also become impure (Levi. 13.11). Therefore, the practices of social restrictions as done in the Zion Christian Church are consistent with the practices of the Old Testament. So, people would normally avoid proximity to the impure person to avoid inflicting impurity in their own lives. Therefore, the Zion Christian Church in the practice of these social restrictions is consistent with the biblical principles or even taboos. Similarly, the many circumstances that might have led to the person being impure such as menstruation and miscarriage among women will be avoided by those who are still in a state of purity. Another taboo is unmarried women lusting after married men because it might lead to sexual impurity. Even this taboo is consistent with the biblical principles of avoiding sexual intercourse with a married person as it would lead to sexual impurity (Levi. 20.10). In the Zion Christian Church, such women would be prevented from coming into close contact, for example, with the livestock in the kraal or even on the farm because it could lead to the death of the livestock or non-productivity in farming. Therefore, in cleansing all these conditions that might result from taboos, there is a need to apply certain healing rituals; hence, taboos and social restrictions are part of the ritual healing process. It is also important to point out that the observance of many of these taboos and social restrictions is consistent with biblical practices, particularly the Old Testament. As Cabrita (2018:16) states, the Zion Christian Church and other African Independent Churches are relevant for the understanding of purity and holiness codes.

The previous chapters, particularly Chapter 2, pointed to the influence of John Alexander Dowie in the Zion Christian Church. Dowie owned land, where he planned to have a lifestyle characterized by holiness and different from other lifestyles in the cities. Dowie established various businesses that would also be different from many other businesses in cities across the globe. It is important to point out that the practices of taboos and social restrictions were part of Zion City that Dowie planned to build in Illinois. Dowie envisaged a city of holiness that would be achieved by placing social restrictions on the members of his church. According to Morton (2013:2):

> He established a theocratic political and economic structure and prohibited smoking, drinking, eating pork, and the practice of any form of modern medicine. He also established a range of businesses, healing homes, and a large Tabernacle. Followers from across the world descended on Zion.

In following Dowie's teachings, the Zion Christian Church also envisaged to have social restrictions and taboos imposed on their members (Hollenweger & MacRobert 1988:44). Moria was specifically built like Zion City in Illinois, where the members of the church would be restricted from eating certain foods and behaving in certain ways. In this way, Zion City was more like Moria in keeping the church to live a life separate and different from the rest of society. Like Zion City, Moria implemented social restrictions and taboos as part of the ritual healing process not only to keep the members of the church holy but also to invoke healing or well-being in their lives (Kruger & Saayman 2016). Therefore, both Zion City in Illinois and Moria in South Africa can be discussed in the context of the ritual healing process in maintaining social restrictions. Here we see a strong connection between American Zionism and South African Zionism and not necessarily the connections between African Independent Churches and traditional African religions as scholars such as Sundkler (1961), Hanekom (1975) and Mokgobi (2014) have suggested.

In keeping the taboos, the Zion Christian Church is keeping up with societal expectations. In other words, the taboos and social restrictions in the Zion Christian Church are kept as part of African cosmology, African mythology and African culture. In the next sections, it will be seen that many of the taboos are practised even outside the precinct of spirituality. These taboos are kept as part of the indigenous practices and not only spiritual practices. Moripe (1998:2) explains, 'In the African Zionist case, the prescriptions and taboos of everyday life are part of the order of meaningful actions which seek to intervene in the contradictory relationship between local people and the larger system that contains them. As in many reformist movements, dietary prescriptions are important signifiers of the reconstructed life in Zion.' However, we can argue that the taboos and restrictions in the Zion Christian Church go beyond cultural observation and have spiritual meaning, particularly when we look at them through the lens of the ritual healing process. This is because the members of the church would know that missing a taboo does not only have consequences in terms of cultural expectations in African society but also the well-being of an individual. But it must be pointed out that the connections between social restrictions to African culture do not result in the connections between traditional African religion and the Zion Christian Church.

The Zion Christian Church and social distancing during the Covid-19 pandemic

The novel coronavirus disease 2019 (Covid-19) started in Wuhan, China, as a cluster of pneumonia cases. Severe acute respiratory syndrome coronavirus 2 (SARS-CoV-2) causes Covid-19, according to the World Health Organization (WHO) (2022). On 5 March 2020, the first case was reported in South Africa of a 38-year-old man who had traveled overseas together with his wife. It was around this time that Covid-19 started spreading across the globe and became a contagious disease affecting many people. Given the spread of Covid-19 in the first quarter of 2020, on 23 March 2020 (almost twenty days after the first case was reported in South Africa), President Cyril Ramaphosa announced a total shutdown of the economy (also known as lockdown) that became effective from 26 March 2020. According to Ozili (2020:1), restrictive measures that were imposed to control the spread of the disease included:

> [R]estricting non-essential activities, closing schools and universities, encouraging people to stay home, lockdown entire cities, requiring essential businesses to run skeletal operations and employees should work from home.

With this kind of restrictions, it meant that even churches had to close given the hard lockdown where everyone was expected to stay indoors and not go out, including to prayer meetings. It is important to note that during this time, a vaccine for Covid-19 had not yet been explored; hence, it was pivotal for governments around the world to put their citizens in a total lockdown and implement the total shutdown of the economy in the same way that President Ramaphosa did in South Africa. This was necessary to control the spread of the disease from one person to the next; hence, those who were infected were isolated for the same purpose.

The Zion Christian Church was one of the first churches to accept the restrictions imposed by the government of South Africa on the churches during the hard lockdown in March 2020. Bishop B. E. Lekganyane, together with the council of his office, read the following statement:

> We would like to let you know that from the weekend of 21 to 22 March, the church choir and (*mekhukhu*), who were supposed to help with the church service preparations on the weekend of 28 to 29 March 2020, along with the Sunday school members and all church singers, that they should not come to Moria until further notice. We appeal that you obey our instructions and wait for further instructions from Moria. We hope that you will peacefully accept our notice. (Sibanyoni 2020:1)

After this statement by the Bishop, the church announced that they were postponing the annual Easter conference in 2020. The reason for the postponement was because of the social restrictions that the government had placed on churches that year. The church made this important decision to save lives by avoiding the spread of the virus from one church member to the next. Even though the church is very strong on ritual healing, they did not want to risk many lives because their Easter gatherings were well attended by people from different parts of the world. Therefore, the risks of meeting during the Covid-19 pandemic were very high. Many lives would have been lost if the church was not proactive in calling off the conference. Many people, including President Ramaphosa, thanked the church for being considerate and closing during the hard lockdown. This should be understood in the context of the church's great knowledge of social restrictions as part of the ritual healing process. Moreover, this does not in any way bring the church closer to traditional African medicine whereby some of the traditional healers insisted on continuing with their practices even during Covid-19.

The Zion Christian Church remained closed during Level 3 of the lockdown, despite President Ramaphosa announcing that small religious gatherings would be allowed when the country went from Level 4 to Level 3 from 1 June 2020. According to Mosia (2022:1), this was an important thing for the church to do given that Covid-19 claimed the lives of many people in South Africa and elsewhere in the world. The church did not claim to have a cure for the virus but rather opted to keep their congregants and others safe by maintaining social distancing during the lockdown. It was important for the church to remain closed given their large following; therefore, this could have led to many fatalities. At this point, only small churches managed to have fellowship. Again, we see the church being considerate of its members and South Africans at large by ensuring that the church remained closed during the hard lockdowns. This means that the social restrictions that were implemented, such as social distancing, during the hard lockdowns remained an important factor for the church even when the government allowed fellowship. This is because the Zion Christian Church is very strong on social restrictions and taboos; hence, it was easy for the church to keep their doors closed even when the government said they could open them. This means that the Covid-19 lockdowns and the social restrictions thereof can be discussed in the context of the ritual healing process, particularly in observing the lockdown rules to keep their members healthy during the pandemic. This is even more pronounced in the church remaining closed even when the government of South Africa allowed churches to have fellowship in small numbers.

The church remained closed as the government kept on decreasing the level of the hard lockdown until the social distancing and the state of national disaster were lifted. Bishop Lekganyane released a statement saying that it was not yet safe to resume the services of the Zion Christian Church. He announced that the churches would stay closed until further notice despite the green light from the government. It was only in 2024 that the Zion Christian Church's headquarters opened its doors for the Easter conference after four years of not having the

Easter conference or any other conference. This was a special year for the church, as they were celebrating the centenary of the inception of the church in 1924. Hence, again, thousands of members of the Zion Christian Church traveled from different corners of the world to attend the Easter conference after years of no celebration due to Covid-19 rules and regulations. Therefore, one can conclude that social distancing was related to the social restrictions of the Zion Christian Church and therefore part of the ritual healing process. The church could implement the restrictions of the hard lockdown given their idea of social restrictions and taboos. This knowledge in the Zion Christian Church became important during the pandemic. However, this knowledge of social restrictions and taboos cannot be linked with traditional African medicine.

The Zion Christian Church and food taboos

The Zion Christian Church follows the Old Testament laws that prohibit eating certain animals. Although writing from a Nigerian context, Chukwuma (2022) highlights these Jewish dietary laws that many African Independent Churches have come to practice when reading the Old Testament. The members of the Zion Christian Church, particularly those who have been baptized, are not permitted to eat pork (Moripe 1998:3). Deuteronomy 14.8 states very well, 'And the swine, because it divideth the hoof, yet cheweth not the cud, it is unclean unto you: ye shall not eat of their flesh, nor touch their dead carcass.' Therefore, the Zion Christian Church prohibits the eating of pork based on the biblical text in the Old Testament. In addition, in the Zion Christian Church, the animals that are prohibited from being eaten must not even be mentioned by name in the church by its members or followers (Moripe 1998:1). This brings a connection between the dietary laws and the taboos, as it is a taboo to mention prohibited food. Concerning the prohibition of pork, it does not matter whether it is the domestic one or the wild one; they are all prohibited. Therefore, both pigs are considered impure, and the baptized members of the Zion Christian Church are not to eat it. However, the state of impurity of the pig is not the only reason why the pig is prohibited in the Zion Christian Church; the other reason is that the totem for the Lekganyane family is 'pig.' Therefore, the family members cannot eat a pig, as it is their totem; consequently, this taboo was extended to the members of the church. In some families the killing of such an animal would result in repercussions; hence, many people in Africa are careful not to do so. Here, we see mainly familial food taboo that is becoming an ecclesiastical food taboo because of the influence of the Lekganyane family in the Zion Christian Church. Nonetheless, the biblical rationale for not eating pork remains the main reason. This demonstrates the connections between the practices of social restrictions in the Zion Christian Church and the Old Testament. This also in a way implies that there are disconnections between traditional African medicine and the church when it comes to social restrictions.

In the Zion Christian Church, edible food is pure food and healthy for the body. Therefore, any food that is not pure and considered to be unhealthy for the body is not permitted in the church. This means that even in the Old Testament, the food that is not edible on the Jewish dietary list is considered not healthy (Chukwuma 2022:2). Chukwuma (2022:3) explains further:

> The food laws were meant to control the dietary behaviors of the people chosen by God. The Ten Commandments were silent on issues that pertain to diet; hence, God gave further instructions that would ensure that the Israelites did not become contaminated by what they consumed. Old Testament dietary laws are mainly documented in Leviticus 11 and 17.

Therefore, the church is consistent with the instructions in Leviticus in keeping up with the social restrictions. The Zion Christian Church also perceives certain diets as not proper and healthy for their members. There are other foods that the members of the Zion Christian Church are not expected to eat in keeping with the church laws and taboos. One such food is Mopani worms, which even though they are readily available (particularly in Limpopo province), the majority of baptized members of the church do not eat. This is not the same as many classical Pentecostal churches that would have this kind of diet. Similarly, many Africans – even those practising traditional African religions – would eat these kinds of food. Therefore, we see a discontinuity between traditional African medicine and the Zion Christian church when it comes to the food that is not considered edible. This, therefore, demonstrates some disconnections between the traditional African religions and the African Independent Churches.

The social restrictions apply to all members of the church, but they are non-negotiable for the ministers in the Zion Christian Church. Lukhaimane (1980:76) points out that if the minister eats food prepared by a woman who is expecting a baby, they would be required to abstain from serving the people in the church. Moripe (1998:5) explains, 'A minister is not supposed to eat food prepared by or live with a woman who has just given birth. The implication for this practice was that most of the ministers became polygamists, for this would enable them to stay with another wife while serving the church.' In addition, a minister is not allowed to eat food served by a woman during her menstrual cycle; this also is a taboo. Lukhaimane (1980:77) states: 'Such women were not allowed to greet men by shaking hands. If they attended Church services, they did not mix with the congregation, but they usually sat aside. At businesses owned by Zionists, such women were not allowed to work until after seven days.' This kind of prohibition was taken from Levi. 12.1-5, which states:

> And the Lord spake unto Moses, saying Speak unto the children of Israel, saying, If a woman has conceived seed, and born a man child: then she shall be unclean seven days; according to the days of the separation for her infirmity shall she be unclean. And on the eighth day, the flesh of his foreskin shall be circumcised. And she shall then continue in the blood of her purifying three and thirty days; she shall touch no hallowed thing, nor come into the sanctuary until the days of her purifying be fulfilled. But if she bears a maid child, then she shall be unclean two weeks, as in her separation: and she shall continue in the blood of her purifying threescore and six days.

Again, here we see that the practices in the Zion Christian Church regarding social restrictions and taboos are consistent with the Bible. As pointed out several times in this book, this further disconnects the social restrictions in the Zion Christian Church with traditional African medicine.

Purity codes for women

There are purity codes for women in the Zion Christian Church that might not apply to men. Generally, men are considered to be clean, as opposed to women who because of biological changes in their bodies are considered unclean. This would explain the rationale for treating women differently in the church; it does not immediately translate to discrimination but observance of social restrictions for the good of these women. In other words, as will be shown in the rest of this section, there are purity codes for women that do not apply to men. The women in the Zion Christian Church are expected to dress modestly and not expose their bodies. It is easier to wear the church uniform, which automatically makes women presentable than if they wore their clothes. However, even without the church uniform, women are expected to look decent when they are in the church or among others in their local communities. When women feel that they are not dressed appropriately, they should find a cloth to cover their bodies so that they are presentable. Women in Africa are expected to dress appropriately as part of culture, particularly when attending important events such as funerals or weddings. In some villages, when a woman is considered to be dressed inappropriately, she will normally not be allowed to attend a funeral, let alone enter a graveyard. This is sometimes a challenge for modern women in cities who struggle to adapt when visiting villages for funerals. Therefore, the issue of dress codes for women as preserved in the Zion Christian Church its more a cultural thing than a religious thing. It is not a ground to bring connections between African Independent churches and traditional African religions the way scholars such as Sundkler (1961), Hanekom (1975) and Mokgobi (2014) have done.

Women in the Zion Christian Church are expected to cover their heads. Mosupyoe (1999:164) points out, 'The girls and women are taught to respect their bodies by wearing long skirts and dresses, cover their heads with scarves, especially during church.' If a woman is found not to comply with these rules and regulations, she will not be allowed in the church service. Thus, normally, the elderly women teach their girls how to obey the church rules and regulations to avoid embarrassment in front of others during the church service. The practices such as women covering their heads are also taken from 1 Corinthians 11.6, which states: 'If a woman does not cover her head, she should have her hair cut off. And if it is shameful for a woman to have her hair cut or shaved off, she should cover her head.' Consequently, in the Zion Christian Church, women cover their heads as part of the church uniform. However, even when they are not wearing a church uniform, they will find a way to cover their heads not only in respect of the church laws but also to avoid falling sick as a result of not obeying the restrictions. Although men do wear the church cap as part of the church uniform, they do not need to cover their heads because they are perceived to be the heads of their families and not women. Here, we see connections between the practices of the social restrictions in the Zion Christian Church and the New Testament. This in my view proves that the church is more consistent with the Christian practices than with the practices in the traditional African religions. These practices are performed in the Zion Christian Church as part of the ritual healing process because those who do not follow the rules might face illnesses.

The social restrictions and taboos in the Zion Christian Church are part of maintaining sexual purity among the women and to a certain extent the men. Cabrita (2018:11) states that 'Zion taught converts that the radical disciplines of personal holiness made identical demands on women and men, and called for women to forsake fathers, husbands, and brother in pursuit of Christian purity'. As pointed out earlier, it is taboo for single women to lust after married men, as it might lead to sexual impurity. This is consistent with the prohibition of sexual intercourse with married partners which alone can bring sickness and diseases. This does not only apply to women alone but equally, men are also prohibited to have sexual intercourse with married women as per the Old Testament. Therefore, in the Zion Christian church both men and women are expected to observe these social restrictions to avoid sexual impurity which leads to sexual illness and diseases. However, it must be pointed out that some restrictions would apply to women because of the biological changes that exist in their bodies such as the menstrual cycle which do not exist in men. This should never be interpreted as a form of discrimination as some scholars such as Mosupyoe (1999) have done. The point in this book is that the Zion Christian Church borrows from the Bible in the practice of these social restrictions rather than the traditional African religions. This argument is made against scholars such as Sundkler (1961), Hanekom (1975) and Mokgobi (2014) who have drawn parallelism between African Independent Churches like the Zion Christian Church and the traditional African religions.

The women in the Zion Christian Church are not expected to touch the healing rituals carried by ministers, particularly the brown paper and other paper strips used to heal the people in the church (Wouters 2014). If a woman touches the healing rituals, she would have to be cleansed by the minister to avoid possible illness because of impurity. In addition, women are not allowed to touch the church uniform of men, as discussed in Chapter 4. If they do so, it is considered a taboo and can lead to sickness and disease. As a result, in the Zion Christian Church, men are expected to wash and iron their uniforms to avoid afflictions on their wives or any other woman. Therefore, women face two difficulties: becoming impure when touching men's attire and imposing impurity upon men when men touch their attire. It is implied that women are considered unclean in many ways in the Zion Christian Church, even when it is not through their actions but those of their male counterparts. Even when men wash their uniforms, they add some drops of water into the bucket so that if a woman by chance touches their clothes, they will still become clean. However, these differences should be understood in the context of purity and impurity, not necessarily in the context of discrimination against women. In addition, these social restrictions are connected with the principles of purity and impurity in the Old Testament.

It must be reiterated that women's uncleanness is based on their biological changes such as menstrual cycles, pregnancy, abortions and complications in their bodies. Women who are in a menstrual circle are considered impure for seven days. This means that for that time, they are restricted in their interactions with others in the church. For example, if a woman in her menstrual cycle attends church, she will be expected to keep away from others to avoid sickness and disease on others. Consequently, to avoid any challenge, women in their menstrual cycle rather opt to stay away from the church for fear of inflicting others because of their uncleanness. It is important to point out that men do not face the same challenges because they do not go through these biological changes. Hence, women are considered to be more unclean than men. Consequently, women are not allowed to touch healing rituals, as discussed above, because of these biological changes, but they would generally be allowed to drink tea to remain pure. This is to ensure that women experiencing some form of impurity are cleansed through the purification rituals.

It is not only menstruating women who are not allowed to attend church. Women who have just given birth are not allowed to attend the church service as they too are considered to be unclean. I have observed while a member of the Zion Christian Church that the woman is expected to stay away for three to six months until other women come to pray with her to release her from the maternity bed. This ceremony is common in the Zion Christian Church and is called *go entsa ngwana* in Northern Sotho, which is loosely translated as the ceremony of 'releasing the child' who has just been born. These are some of the challenges that women face in the Zion Christian Church. However, in my observation, the women in this church do not necessarily view these kinds of treatment as part of discrimination but as part of helping them to undergo the ritual healing process to maintain their well-being. Therefore, even when literature and scholarship demonstrate the negative sides of the purity codes for women, the women do not see it that way. Therefore, the purity codes for women in the Zion Christian Church are part of the ritual healing process and linked to the Christian practices in the Old Testament as opposed to linking them with traditional African religions.

No smoking and drinking

Generally, the members of the Zion Christian Church do not drink alcohol or smoke tobacco. In the African Independent Churches, alcohol and tobacco are perceived as coming from the devil (Strohbehn 2016:278). Similarly, most of the Pentecostal churches in Africa do not drink alcohol and do not smoke tobacco. The baptized members of the Zion Christian Church are expected to maintain high levels of morals, which include not drinking and smoking. This also means that the members of the church would not be found in beer halls, taverns, bottle stores, and other drinking and smoking spaces. Generally, the prohibition of smoking and drinking among church members is emphasized during the baptism. Again, it is important to point out that these restrictions are viewed as part of the ritual healing process. Because the members of the Zion Christian Church abstain from these practices, they are more likely to be healthy than most people who use smoking and alcohol. According to the World Health Organisation (2022:1): 'Drinking alcohol is associated with risks of developing non-communicable diseases such as liver diseases, heart diseases, and different types of cancers, as well as mental health and behavioral conditions such as depression, anxiety, and alcohol use disorders.' Similarly, Marks (2012:73) states: 'Smokers increase their risk of lung disease, including lung cancer. But they also increase their risk of other illnesses such as heart disease, stroke, and mouth (oral) cancer. Risks from smoking, as they relate to lung disease, include the Chronic obstructive pulmonary disease (COPD).' Therefore, time and again, the members of the Zion Christian Church are encouraged to stop smoking and drinking as this has a bearing on their health. The church members are usually encouraged to drink the tea prepared by the pastors, as discussed in Chapter 3, which in a way replaces the drinking of alcohol and the smoking of tobacco.

The ministers of the church are expected to keep this restriction, as it has a bearing on the healing rituals in the Zion Christian Church. Moripe (1998:4) explains, 'If a preacher, deacon or minister smokes or drinks, his certificate should be confiscated and he should cease his duties as an ordained leader forthwith.' The same standards are upheld among the pastors in the Pentecostal and charismatic churches in Africa, with pastors expected not to drink and smoke or their licenses will be revoked. While some members of the church (particularly recovering addicts of smoking or drinking) may be tempted to drink and smoke again, they will not do so in their church uniform or while wearing a badge. Lukhaimane (1980:73) explains, 'It was known amongst the members that no person would dare drink or smoke with a badge on because the non-members would remark on this and even reject him.' Therefore, even when there is a failure in terms of obeying the church's restrictions on smoking and drinking, the expectations are that it should not be done when wearing the church uniform to avoid defiling the uniform. However, the main reason for not smoking or drinking remains the quest to be healthy to live long as part of the healing ritual processes in the Zion Christian Church. This explains why the members of the church would obey and refrain from drinking alcohol and smoking tobacco. This connects the church with a healthy lifestyle within the framework of the ritual healing process. The quest for the church to live a healthy lifestyle has nothing to do with the traditional African religions which again makes it impossible for the links with the latter. On the contrary, observing non-alcoholism and non-smoking are practices encouraged in the Old Testament as Levi. 10.9 states 'You and your sons are not to drink wine or strong drink when you enter the Tent of Meeting, or else you will die; this is a permanent statute for the generations to come.' Therefore, the Zion Christian Church is very much consistent with the Christian practices as laid out in the Old Testament.

Restrictions during death and funerals

Death and funerals are also part of the restrictions and taboos within the Zion Christian Church. This is also part of African cosmology, where taboos and rules are defined in terms of life in the now and in death, funerals and the afterlife (Olupona 2014). Moripe (1998:1) points out that in the Zion Christian Church, anything that has to do with death is considered taboo. This includes the restrictions on touching the dead, being around the dead or anything around the dead, including belongings of the dead. In some instances, these include restrictions on naming the dead or anything associated with the name of the dead. The clothes of the dead cannot be shared among the living without a proper prayer that necessitates the cleansing of the belongings. In some instances, even touching the corpse necessitates some cleansing, as those who have done so are considered to be impure. In the Zion Christian Church, these restrictions are considered taboos and should be observed by the church members. If the church member has contact with death due to the passing of a family member or attending a funeral service, they are required to stay away from the church for seven days until they are cleansed. This means that for every funeral attended by a baptized church member, they would have to miss at least one Sunday service to be cleansed before attending the church service again. Anderson (2000:213) notes: 'The bereaved should stay at home, should not socialise or have sexual contact or even go to church.' This practice in the Zion Christian Church is consistent with the Old Testament. Numbers 19.11-13 'Whoever touches a human corpse will be unclean for seven days. They must purify themselves with the water on the third day and on the seventh day; then they will be clean. But if they do not purify themselves on the third and seventh days, they will not be clean. If they fail to purify themselves after touching a human corpse, they defile the LORD's tabernacle. They must be cut off from Israel. Because the water of cleansing has not been sprinkled on them, they are unclean; their uncleanness remains on them.' It is for this reason that anyone who attends a funeral should be sprinkled with water afterwards, and ministers would be required to stay away from the church for seven days as discussed below.

The restrictions on death, funerals and the afterlife are applied rigidly when it comes to the ministers of the Zion Christian Church. According to Moripe (1998:5), 'Ministers of the [Zion Christian Church] have strict rules of purification, for example, they are not allowed to pray for a sick person if they have attended a funeral.' This means that the cleansing mechanism applied to the church members on death and at funerals also applies to the ministers of the church. These ministers would have to stay away from the church for about seven days after which they would be allowed to minister again. This period provides an opportunity for the minister or the pastor of the church to be cleansed from being in contact with the dead, death or funerals. According to Lukhaimane (1980:56), this makes the ministers very careful when attending funerals for fear of being impure. As a result, some of the ministers in the Zion Christian Church would rather opt for staying away from funerals to remain pure and be able to minister to the church members. This is a challenge because the same ministers are supposed to pray for people after they attend the funerals, as discussed in Chapter 3 of this book. Therefore, the pastors of the Zion Christian Church are always in the middle of the road between the fear of being impure and the ritual of cleansing others during funerals. Consequently, it is sometimes not their choice, but they go to funerals as per the scheduling of the church leadership in local branches. Hence, it is common in these branches for the pastors to rotate attendance of funerals to avoid having all the pastors not attending church because of their impurity. In addition, it must be reiterated that this is in keeping up with the instructions in Numbers 19 to avoid impurity which might result in sickness and diseases.

The restrictions and taboos on death also mean that anyone present during death is considered unclean. For example, if a member of the church dies in a car accident, those with whom would also be considered unclean, particularly if they are also members of the church. Hence, in the Zion Christian Church, cleansing from death involves going to the site where the death occurred and being able to cleanse those who were involved in the death. Even when the death happens at home, the expectation is that the pastors should immediately go and pray with the family as part of the cleansing ceremony and the healing practice of the bereaved family. Hence, it is a practice in the Zion Christian Church for the members of the church to support fellow members through prayer during funerals as part of the ritual healing process. Therefore, the kind of death that the family suffers contributes to the uncleanness of those who are around them. It is also important to mention that this is part of the ritual healing process because the lack of cleansing might result in the death of those who are still alive in the family. This also explains the reason why the members of the Zion Christian Church dedicate their cars so that they are exempted from accidents in the first place. However, since accidents happen anyway, they would avoid misfortune and conduct various cleansing ceremonies at the accident sites. The observance of the social restriction when it comes to death, burials and funerals is observed in the Zion Christian Church as per the Old Testament and therefore should be separated from observances in the traditional African religions.

The unveiling of tombstones

One way in which the dead are respected within African cosmology is by erecting a tombstone next to or on the grave of the dead. The erection of tombstones cannot be separated from other rituals, including burial rituals. There are several reasons why Africans would erect and unveil a tombstone as part of the rituals of death. Kgatle and Mashau (2023:3) state:

> The erection of a tombstone and its unveiling is meant to mark the grave and serves as an act of achieving closure by the family – closure from life in this world to ancestry and the spiritual world. The unveiling of a tombstone also marks the end of the mourning period. Second, the ritual/ceremony serves as a memorial event. It allows family members to celebrate the deceased's life by remembering all of their good deeds.

In addition, the erection of the tombstone is done as a sign of respecting the dead and in a quest to commemorate the dead. The tombstones may be erected during the funeral or in a separate ceremony. The reason for this is that the erection of the tombstone has become an expansive exercise that requires a serious budget. Hence, some families can do it on the day of the funeral, while others need a separate ceremony. Nonetheless, even after the erection of the tombstone, there would be a ceremony to unveil the tombstone of the dead to which family members and relatives would be invited. According to Harrington (2022), a ceremony like this would require the sacrifice of either a cow or a lamb as part of the ritual of unveiling the tombstone.

The taboos and social restrictions imposed on the members of the Zion Christian Church during the death and funerals of their loved ones would also apply when it comes to the ceremony of unveiling the tombstones. In my observation, many of the African Independent Churches would not restrict their members from attending or even conducting ceremonies concerning the unveiling of tombstones. Many of these churches would not discourage their members from attending these ceremonies. Similarly, in the Zion Christian Church, the members of the church attend the unveiling of tombstones. In this church, the ceremony of unveiling a tombstone is considered an important one, in the same way as when the bereaved family buries their loved one. Therefore, members are not necessarily restricted from attending such ceremonies. However, in the Zion Christian Church, when one attends such ceremonies, they are considered impure and kept away from the church for seven days to receive cleansing in the same way as when one has attended a funeral. Hence, some members of the Zion Christian Church would shy away from attending the unveiling of tombstone ceremonies so that they could remain pure. As discussed in the previous sections, it is even more difficult for the ministers of the church, as they are required to remain pure for ministry. Therefore, attending an unveiling of the tombstone ceremony would require the minister to undergo cleansing before they can minister to the church members again. Again, this is discussed in the context of the ritual healing process, as non-observance of the restrictions and taboos would lead to illnesses. In addition, one can point out that in the unveiling ceremonies as is the case with funerals, the Zion Christian Church observes the social restrictions and rules as stipulated in the Old Testament particularly Numbers 19. This means that the unveiling ceremony like the funeral ceremony as practised in the Zion Christian Church is more consistent with the Christian faith than the traditional African religions.

Initiation schools

Initiation is the rite of passage within African culture that is meant to mark acceptance into manhood or womanhood (Ikwuagwu 2006). Therefore, in many tribes, to demonstrate that one has grown into manhood or womanhood, one would be initiated through an initiation school. In most tribes, men would be expected to go to an initiation school in the mountains for four to six weeks, depending on the practice of a specific school. For women, the initiation school can take place even at home, where elderly women would be expected to initiate a young woman into adulthood. Therefore, initiation can be defined as the process of transforming a girl or a boy into a new role of responsibility in African society. Brown (2012:123) explains that circumcision is the ritual conducted as part of the initiation ritual marking a graduation from childhood to adulthood. It was also conducted in biblical times, as stated in Gen. 17.12-24:

> And he that is eight days old shall be circumcised among you, every man child in your generations, he that is born in the house, or bought with money of any stranger, which is not of thy seed. He that is born in thy house, and he that is bought with thy money, must needs be circumcised: and my covenant shall be in your flesh for an everlasting covenant. And the uncircumcised man child whose flesh of his foreskin is not circumcised, that soul shall be cut off from his people; he hath broken my covenant.

Therefore, it appears that circumcision in the biblical context was done as part of sealing a covenant with God. It is a bit different from the practice of circumcision in the traditional African religions, where there are also different rituals performed as part of the initiation ceremonies.

The Zion Christian Church is not necessarily opposed to the idea of being circumcised but rather to the various traditional African religious rituals conducted as part of the initiation school. There is a distinction between circumcision (*lebollo* in Northern Sotho) and initiation (*koma*). Initiation has some implications of being initiated into different rituals within traditional African religions. Consequently, in the Zion Christian Church, the boys and the girls are not encouraged to go to initiation schools. It is worse if the baptized member of the Zion Christian Church visited the initiation school, as they would not be allowed to attend church for the duration of the initiation. Hence, I observed that many members of the Zion Christian Church take their children away to other places where there is no initiation school, particularly during winter, to prevent them from attending it. Therefore, the members of the Zion Christian Church are always caught between observing the church's restrictions on initiation schools and the African culture or expectations of children to be initiated. I need to point out that in my observation, the children of the members of the Zion Christian Church end up attending initiation schools as the pressure from society to be initiated as boys and girls exceeds that of the church regarding the restrictions on initiation schools. In other words, there is a stigma attached to people who are not initiated, even if some are circumcised by medical doctors. In the end, even if they are members of the Zion Christian Church, they end up being initiated and suffer the consequences of not attending church later.

The good thing is that attendance at initiation school does not make one lose membership in the Zion Christian Church but only restricts church attendance, which is bearable. Nonetheless, the restrictions on initiation schools demonstrate some disconnections with the traditional African religions.

The sacrality and centrality of Moria

Moria is the headquarters of the Zion Christian Church, as discussed in Chapter 3 of this book. It is named after the biblical name for Jerusalem in 2 Chron. 3.1, 'Then Solomon began to build the temple of the Lord in Jerusalem on Mount Moriah, where the Lord had appeared to his father David. It was on the threshing floor of Araunah[a] the Jebusite, the place provided by David.' So, in calling the headquarters Moria, the Zion Christian Church once again uses the Old Testament for its Christian practices. In addition, they contextualize their headquarters in a significant manner, similar to that of Jerusalem. Thus, Moria becomes the Jerusalem of the adherents of the Zion Christian Church. Therefore, Moria as the headquarters of the Zion Christian Church is not an ordinary place but rather a sacred place where members and followers expect to receive healing. Moria is perceived as a holy place that is quite distinct from other places. Therefore, people do not go to Moria for tourism or entertainment purposes but they do so to receive the blessing bestowed by the Bishop. Lukhaimane (1980:35) explains, 'Members came to Moria to receive strength in their faith and blessings from the "Messiah". The members of the church believed that when visiting Moria, it was a place where they would hear God speak through the mouth of the bishop. Thus, some staunch believers would roll down where Engenas had passed because they believed they would be healed or blessed.' Unlike the sanctuary in the local branches of the Zion Christian Church, Moria is considered very sacred and a place that contains the blessing of the Lord through the servant of the Lord, the Bishop. For many members of the church, Moria is a sacred place where they not only worship God but also expect to receive the blessing of the Lord. It is for the same reason that, as discussed previously, many would flock to Moria during the Easter conference and other important meetings organized by the Zion Christian Church in the quest to receive the same blessings.

Moria also helps the church in terms of centrality and ability to bring all the members of the church into one central place. Anderson (1999:306) points out that 'the emphasis on the powerful central headquarters at Moria to which members are expected to converge, and the ultimate authority of the bishop in all areas of church activities in the outlying branches, has resulted in the Zion Christian Church being able to avoid the abundance of secessions that has characterized so many other African Independent Churches.' This means that even though the church has grown to greater numbers, the centre holds, which is the headquarters of the church – Moria. The centrality of the headquarters also becomes the foundation of the centrality of the church leaders, such as Engenas Lekganyane, Edward Lekganyane and Barnabas Lekganyane. Therefore, the members of the church always look forward to visiting Moria and seeing their bishop(s) as part of the ritual healing process. Thus, touching the headquarters and walking where the bishop walked became part of the healing ritual for many members of the Zion Christian Church. Moreover, according to Lukhaimane (1980:16), many members of the church believe that each time they visit Moria, it must be windy – which symbolizes the presence of God in that place. Therefore, in a way, Moria is the dwelling place of God, similar to the way that New Jerusalem is believed to be the dwelling place of God. The point made here is that Moria is not an ordinary place; it serves as a sanctuary and a place where members of the church believe they will receive their healing upon arrival in Moria. Therefore, the Zion Christian Church's headquarters form part of the ritual healing process. In addition, Moria should be defined as the place where all the restrictions discussed in this chapter are epitomized. This means that Moria becomes a place where food such as pork is not allowed; where purity codes for women are observed; where there is no smoking of tobacco and drinking of alcohol; and where restrictions during death, funerals and the unveiling of tombstones are observed. It is a place where initiation schools are not allowed. It is a holy place. This place practices social restrictions as per the instructions in Num. 19, not necessarily the practices of the traditional African religions as argued by scholars like Sundkler (1961), Hanekom (1975) and Mokgobi (2014). This is how the Zion Christian Church and other African Independent Churches have shaped the religious landscape in Africa because of instilling the holiness principles within the context of the ritual healing process (Cabrita 2018:6).

Conclusion

This chapter discussed the social restrictions and taboos in the Zion Christian Church that have therapeutic and protective implications in the life of the believer or members of this church. The church has many taboos, which in a way contribute to the well-being of the believers in the Zion Christian Church. It is for the same reason that the Zion Christian Church was the first to agree to the government's measures of social distancing during the Covid-19 pandemic. One kind of taboo or restriction in the Zion Christian Church is on food, particularly the prohibition on eating pork and animals that died of illness. The women in this church are expected to dress respectfully for their well-being. Smoking and drinking are discouraged, particularly among the church ministers as a measure not only of social restrictions but also of holiness. Other restrictions exist in the church concerning death, how funerals should be conducted and how members should behave during such ceremonies. There are also restrictions concerning the unveiling of tombstones of the members of the church. The members of the church whose children have attended initiation schools are not supposed to go to church for a certain number of weeks. The headquarters of the Zion Christian Church itself is considered a sacred place with many restrictions, particularly for visitors because prior permission is required before visiting the site. These social restrictions and taboos were discussed as part of the ritual healing process. It was found that social restrictions and taboos contribute to the well-being of the members of the Zion Christian Church. The same taboos and social restrictions exist in traditional African medicine, but their practices are not the same as the ritual healing process in the Zion Christian Church. This again brings disconnections between traditional African medicine and healing in the Zion Christian Church when it comes to social restrictions.

8

Distinctive healing in the Zion Christian Church

Introduction

The last chapter is a summary of findings on dissociating traditional African medicine from the ritual healing process in the Zion Christian Churches. The findings are determined by revisiting the various healing, worship, protection, restriction, taboos and prophecy practices to conclude their dissociation with traditional African medicine. However, when making these dissociations, the distinctions between indigenization and syncretism also need to be made clearly. This is important because the indigenization of healing rituals is different from traditional African medicine. It is therefore important to highlight these differences to avoid not only generalizations but also the paganization and demonization of the ritual healing process, not only in the Zion Christian Church but also in the broader spectrum among the African Independent Churches. By using the Zion Christian Church as a case study, the role and development of ritual healing theology in the African Independent Churches can be explored.

Distinct healing rituals in the Zion Christian Church

This book studied the ritual healing process in the Zion Christian Church by identifying the dissociations with traditional African medicine in various healing rituals. With the use of small pieces of wood in the Zion Christian Church, there is a disconnection with traditional African medicine. This practice is disconnected from traditional African medicine because the piece of wood is prayed over by the minister calling the name of the Father, the Son and the Holy Spirit. Ordinarily, in the African traditional religions, sticks would be used calling ancestors and invoking other spirits. The use of blessed tea in the Zion Christian Church, in some way, is connected with the use of different herbal teas within the context of the ritual healing process. Again, it is important to point out that tea like many other healing rituals is first prayed over by the pastor which is different from its use in traditional African medicine. The study also found that water from streams and rivers for healing is also prescribed by the prophets in the Zion Christian Church. Traditional healers do visit streams and rivers; however, the difference lies in how these sites are used in terms of the spirits that are invoked in the sites. The study found that, generally, the shedding of blood includes pricking or cutting human beings' flesh, through the use of razors. This is something that is practised in traditional African medicine, but the difference as discussed in Chapter 3 is the prayer. The study found that ministers in the Zion Christian Church use an enema treatment on children and adults in the process of cleansing. While an enema might be used in traditional African medicine, this would be generally for cleansing purposes which is normally done by some Africans whether religious or not as per the ritual healing process. Another practice is in the use of steam as a healing ritual, for both children and the elderly, but like enema, this is a common ritual of healing within the African context. Therefore, in many healing rituals in the Zion Christian Church, there is a clear disconnection with traditional African medicine.

Furthermore, the study found that there is a dissociation between the practices of protection in the Zion Christian Church and traditional African medicine. The church uniform (*seaparo*) is not worn only for the sake of being appropriately dressed but also serves as a protective measure against attacks of sickness and disease, in a similar way that garments would be used for protection in the military. There is no link between this practice and the traditional African medicine. Practices, such as the sprinkling of water around the house for spiritual protection, are also done in traditional African medicine when Africans seek to protect their homes. However, the difference still lies in the connection between the calling or invoking of spirits within the broader spectrum of traditional African religions. The wearing of the ZCC badge is not only done for church members to identify each other when in public, but it also serves to protect church members against criminals, particularly in urban areas. Another protective healing ritual in the Zion Christian Church is the use of a photograph of the bishop, which is popularly known as *senepe sa mookamedi,* in Northern Sotho. The use of photographs, portraits and artefacts should be seen as forming part of the ritual healing process than as idolization of leaders such as the bishops in the Zion Christian Church. Similarly, the use of strings and strips, which are worn as armour against witchcraft in the Zion Christian Church, is also a common practice within the ritual healing process. In the ritual healing process, it is also common to use copper wires at the gate of one's house for protection against witchcraft and sorcery. The male members of the Zion Christian Church use sticks and whips to protect themselves against any eventuality or mishap while on the road. These practices, that is, strings and strips, copper wires, sticks and whips might be used in traditional African medicine, but the differences lie in their attachments with the spirits in the spirit realm in the latter.

There are some disconnections between worship as a therapeutic tool in the Zion Christian Church and some ceremonies in traditional African medicine. Popular ceremonies such as *mpoho* (ritual prayer) ceremonies, which are performed during the night are distinct from the ceremonies where traditional healers sing for the whole night to invoke ancestral spirits or to initiate an amateur traditional healer. This practice is normally called *malopo* in Northern Sotho. *Mpoho* which is performed by both the male choir and the female choir in the Zion Christian Church is done to engage in spiritual warfare against evil spirits and witchcraft. The fact that both ceremonies (i.e. *mpoho* and *malopo*) are performed at night does not make them similar. Even with the *nkedi* (ZCC dance formation for males), it can be connected to the *Kiba* and the *Dinaka* – traditional song and dance performances in the Bapedi culture but not with the traditional African medicine. The brass band in the Zion Christian Church does not play as part of entertainment but to bring healing among the members and followers of the church which have nothing to do with traditional African medicine. The sermon presentations of the bishops are presented to bring healing and transformation to the congregants rather than just to fulfill liturgical orders. This is disconnected from traditional African medicine since there are no sermons preached in the latter.

There is also a disconnection between prophecy in the Zion Christian Church and divination in traditional African medicine. One of the functions of the prophets *(mabone)* in the Zion Christian Church is to call out members of the church and give them a prophetic word in private, as opposed to in public. Another function of the *mabone* is to trace the cause of the sickness or disease in patients, to provide the relevant prescription. The *mabone* in the Zion Christian Church also knows the events of the future, including the various battles or conflicts between countries. Therefore, bishops, such as Engenas Lekganyane, not only function as the leader of the church but also as the *lebone* (prophet) of the church. The prophet would give instructions and prescriptions to the patient to deal with the root cause of the problem. This phenomenon, known as *ditaelo* (instruction), is important in the Zion Christian Church since it is viewed as a 'do or die' process in the church that members would seldom ignore, for their good. However, we need to differentiate between the prophet in the Zion Christian Church and the diviner in the traditional African religions. The diviner and the prophet would differ when it comes to the source of their divination or prophecy. While the prophet in the Zion Christian Church gives the prophecy by the power of the Holy Spirit, the diviner invokes the power of the other spirits, including ancestral spirits, to receive their revelation. Therefore, prophecy demonstrates some dissociation between the ritual healing process in the Zion Christian Church and traditional African medicine.

Many of the taboo practices in the Zion Christian Church are part of the ritual healing process. One of the taboos or restrictions in the Zion Christian Church is about food, particularly the prohibition on eating pork and animals that died of natural illness. It is also expected of the women in this church to dress respectfully, which is a custom embraced by many Africans. Furthermore, the church discourages smoking and drinking, particularly among the church ministers, not only for social reasons but also as a measure to uphold the command of holiness. Here, again we see a dissociation between the ritual healing process in the Zion Christian Church and the traditional African medicine which would not ordinarily emphasize holiness as a Christian practice. Other restrictions exist in the church concerning death, how funerals should be conducted in the church and how members should behave at such ceremonies. There are restrictions concerning the unveiling of tombstones of the members of the Zion Christian Church, which is also part of the ritual healing process. There are also diverse approaches to initiation, since members of the church, whose children have attended initiation schools, are not supposed to attend church for a certain number of weeks. This is to disconnect the members of the church from the influences that come with initiation in the traditional African religions. The headquarters of the Zion Christian Church, itself, is considered a sacred place, with many restrictions to access, particularly for visitors, where prior permission is required before visiting the site. This again demonstrates the preservation of the church site as a place through which the members and followers of the church can obtain healing. Therefore, most of these healing rituals demonstrate a disconnection with traditional African medicine.

Indigenization of ritual healing process

As highlighted previously, ritual healing in the Zion Christian Church is seen in the practices of healing, prophecy, spiritual protection, worship, taboos and restrictions. In all these aspects of ritual healing in the Zion Christian Church, there seems to be a reliance on the work of the Holy Spirit, particularly in the practice of prophecy. The empowerment of the Holy Spirit is consistent with Christian spirituality, particularly Pentecostal spirituality, as practised by many Pentecostal churches in Africa. Therefore, the reliance on the Holy Spirit for the practice of prophecy in the Zion Christian Church aligns with Christian spirituality. Notably, most of the prophets in the Zion Christian Church speak in tongues, as part of their practice of prophecy, which is a common practice in Africa. However, a closer look at other practices reveals that the church significantly has found creative ways to indigenize healing. As discussed in the preceding sections, there are different healing rituals, such as pieces of wood, holy water, holy tea, pricking, enema and steaming, which are all used as part of indigenous knowledge in the African context. Moreover, the Zion Christian Church uses water that is mixed with sand, as well as copper wires, and strips and strings of cloth. Brown paper, the badge, sticks and whips, and the photograph of the bishop are used for the protection of households and businesses. Furthermore, the members of these churches wear uniforms to protect themselves against witchcraft and sorcery. The different music groups are indiginized in the Zion Christian Church. Unlike in ordinary healing, the Zion Christian Church observes many social restrictions and taboos. These practices might not be common within mainline Christianity but do not immediately become practices of traditional African medicine. The church has found ways in which ordinary indigenous knowledge systems can be infused into the church practices to indiginise Christianity. Therefore, these practices should help us in making distinctions between traditional African medicine and indiginization of the gospel.

In the Zion Christian Church, both Christian and indigenous knowledge are brought together in the practice of ritual healing. For example, the practice of baptism in the church is done in a Christian way through triple immersion. This is something that the church founder, Engenas Lekganyane, replicated from classical Pentecostalism, as the Apostolic Faith Mission also baptizes their members through triple immersion – in the name of the Father, of the Son and of the Holy Spirit. This practice is very much consistent with Christian practices, which are derived from biblical instructions on baptism. However, in the Zion Christian Church, baptism goes beyond the sacramental practices, to act as ritual healing, in the belief that those who are sick can get healed through baptism. Moreover, unlike the classical Pentecostal churches, such as the Apostolic Faith Mission, the Zion Christian Church baptizes the believers in running water, like in a dam or river. The latter is practised by a majority of the African Independent Churches and is consistent with the ritual healing process. Therefore, in sacraments, such as baptism, we see a mixture of Christian practices, particularly in the triple immersion, and observation of ritual healing processes, particularly in the practice of baptism as a healing and deliverance ritual. There are many other examples where we see the mixing of indigenous knowledge systems and Christian practices in the Zion Christian Church. It is, therefore, pivotal to make a distinction between traditional African medicine and the indigenization of the gospel.

The Zion Christian Church is not alone in combining the indigenous knowledge system and Christian practices in the ritual healing process; many other African Independent Churches are known for the same. The African Independent Churches are known for blending indigenous knowledge systems and Christian practices, particularly when it comes to the practice of ritual healing. This very same element has made these churches dynamic, as they appeal to Africans who may seek a ritual healing that embraces both Christian and indigenous knowledge. The Zion Christian Church and other African Independent Churches have done well to have a clear expression and articulation of the customs and traditions in the name of Christianity, to win over both Christians and those who are inclined to indigenous knowledge systems. In the end, both Christian and indigenous knowledge systems are visible in ritual healing in the Zion Christian Church. Hence, the church has been able to attract many adherents, in the African context, as they find the church very attractive and relevant in addressing the many problems that they face. Thus, while churches such as the Zion Christian Church can be critiqued for blending Christian practices with the indigenous knowledge system, it is the same mixture that has made the church popular and contributed to membership. However, we should not mistake this blending as alignment towards traditional African medicine which might lead to the demonization and paganization of African Independent Churches.

Given the clarity between traditional African medicine and indiginization, we cannot immediately perceive certain ritual healing practices to be unchristian or pagan, because many of these practices do not interfere with the Christian faith. To avoid the demonization and paganization of the ritual healing process, it is important to detach from the Western understanding of concepts such as ritual healing into the contextualized understanding of the same. Therefore, this book uses the ritual healing process to contextualize healing in the African Independent Churches. This is a call to understand ritual healing in the context of the African Independent Churches without demonizing the same. This is a call to embrace the ritual healing process even if it is not popular among many mainline Christian churches in Africa.

Theology of ritual healing

The ritual healing process and indigenization of the gospel are important for the development of the theology of ritual healing in African Independent Churches. In the first instance, this theology is developed in the balance between faith healing and the indigenous knowledge system within the ritual healing process. This means that in our theologizing, instead of condemning the Zion Christian Church for using ritual healing, we need to find the intersections of faith healing and indigenous knowledge. These are the intersections of the Christian faith and indigenous knowledge which does not lead to syncretistic practices. As discussed previously, the Zion Christian Church and other African Independent Churches are known for the expression of the Christian faith in the African context. Similarly, the combination of faith healing and indigenous knowledge provides such an expression. This is an important area when studying the theology of ritual healing; we need to find a way of combining both indigenous knowledge and healing rather than approach the two separately. This is important in the understanding of ritual healing not only in the Zion Christian Church but in other African Independent Churches as well.

In the second instance, the theology of ritual healing is developed by making a distinction between its practice in the Zion Christian church and traditional African medicine. This is not a simple matter as there are very thin lines separating the two. This means that ordinarily, traditional African medicine as practised in African Traditional religions can be confused with the ritual healing process in the Zion Christian Church. When the distinctions have been made, it would be possible to see that churches like the Zion Christian Church align with ritual healing but not necessarily with traditional African medicine in African traditional religions. I am not saying this as a judgemental view of the traditional African religions but rather in the context of discussing the Zion

Christian Church as part of local and global Christianity. We need to take note as discussed in the preceding sections about the disconnections, for example, when it comes to the source of prophecy and the source of the remedy that the prophet prescribes to the patient. This is very much different from the source of prophecy and prescription in traditional African medicine. Therefore, the theology of ritual healing should know when it is ritual healing and when it is traditional African medicine. And where there are clear disconnections with traditional African medicine, those should be pointed out.

Third, the theology of ritual healing finds a balance between modern medicine and ritual healing. Some of the African Independent Churches would discourage the use of modern medicine in the name of ritual healing. Some do in some instances discourage the patient from using modern medicine at that moment. Nonetheless, the discouragement of not using modern medicine can be dangerous to some patients leading to deaths. Therefore, a theology of ritual healing is developed by recognizing both modern medicine and ritual healing. This opens up a possibility for one patient to utilize their faith while also not neglecting their modern medicine. In this way, modern medicine is not seen as the enemy of ritual healing but as a complementary type of healing. After all, there are so many modern medicines that have been developed through ritual healing; hence, the two cannot become enemies. Similarly, many health practitioners encourage ritual healing for their patients in addition to the modern medicine given to the patients. Therefore, a development of the theology of ritual healing takes cognizance of both modern medicine and ritual healing. This calls for adherents of churches such as the Zion Christian Church not to be ignorant of the biomedical understanding of sickness and diseases in the name of faith.

The ritual healing theology needs to also be cognizant that the ceremonies, symbols and healing rituals themselves are not the source of healing, but God is the healer. Various biblical texts indicate that God is the one who heals the brokenhearted and those who are wounded (Exod. 15.26, Ps. 147.3, Jer. 3.22). Therefore, God is the one who brings physical, spiritual, emotional and psychological healing. Isaiah 53.5 states very well, 'But he was pierced for our transgressions, he was crushed for our iniquities; the punishment that brought us peace was on him, and by his wounds, we are healed.' In addition, the prophet who is diagnosing the problem of the patient and giving out prescriptions is not the healer, but God is the healer. After all, even with all the healing rituals that a patient can have, there is still a need for the patient to have faith in their healing. Jesus often said to the sick, 'Your faith has made you whole.' In simple terms, Jesus was communicating a message to the sick that it is not pricking, springling, enema, strips, strings copper wire holy water or anything other healing rituals that are important in healing but rather the faith of an individual. James 5:15 states very well, 'And the prayer of faith shall save the sick, and the Lord shall raise him; and if he have committed sins, they shall be forgiven him.' This places the importance of faith in the healing of individuals rather than the rituals themselves. Therefore, the theology of ritual healing in African Independent Churches should not place the rituals ahead of the faith of an individual who is sick.

Implications on African Independent Churches

The African Independent Churches are studied as a movement that broke away from the Western missionary churches given the alignment of the latter with the ecclesiastical polity of the early twentieth century. These churches became popular, at that time, because of their quest to respond to the oppression of Black people in the Western missionary churches. This means that the many Black people, who were part of these Western missionary churches, moved to join the African Independent Churches in solidarity, to free Black people from oppression. This means that African Independent Churches can be studied and understood as the churches that sought freedom from Western administrative and political injustices. In fact, at that time, many Black leaders could not become pastors and were led by white pastors, who were appointed to oversee the Black church. Therefore, in resistance to this kind of oppression and injustice, many African Independent Churches emerged in South Africa and elsewhere on the continent. They sought a spirituality that would not discriminate against them as Black people but would affirm them as part of God's creation. This was not the case in many classical Pentecostal churches, which, at that time, aligned with the political atmosphere and divided the church, instead of uniting it. This, in my view, is what contributed to the proliferation of these churches and how the scholarship on this topic came about – to understand this phenomenon and the rationale behind the growth of the African Independent Churches. It was mainly for the reason that churches that would appeal to Black people were founded, to free Black people from the oppression within the ranks of conventional churches. This puts the African Independent Churches in the same category as the Black consciousness movements that sought the liberation of Black people. Hence, the need to understand this means that these churches, particularly in their early inception, represented the Black majority in the fight for freedom in countries such as South Africa.

However, the African Independent Churches are not only studied as a breakaway movement from the Western missionary churches, but they should also be understood as the churches that sought the indigenization of the gospel, that is, preaching a gospel that is relevant to the African people. This makes the African Independent Churches, together with Pentecostal churches, a movement that can contextualize the gospel in the African context. In other words, these are churches that can present the gospel by using the African indigenous knowledge systems, and they were also able to de-Westernise the gospel – making it more relevant in the African context to the African people. In a way, spiritual practices, such as healing and prophecy, became the tools by which many leaders in the African Independent Churches were able to Africanize the gospel. They use these spiritual experiences to be able to deal with African problems that emanated from the spirit realm, such as witchcraft, misfortune, sorcery and so forth. Because many of these problems are linked to the spiritual realm, many Africans are attracted to the African Independent Churches to be able to address these challenges. The African Independent Churches can be understood as a religious group that sought to bring an alternative to modern medicine by using ritual healing, to deal with challenges that could not be addressed by modern medicine. The African Independent Church is studied as a religious group that can trace the root cause of the problem through the use of both diagnostic prophecy and prescriptive prophecy. The combination of both diagnostic and prescriptive prophecy is used to bring divine healing to believers in the African Independent Churches. Hence, ritual healing in the churches can be studied and understood as the main factor that contributed to the popularity and growth of the African Independent Churches. It can also be understood as the tool that these churches used to mitigate the gaps that the Western missionary churches could not fill among African believers, particularly regarding the link between African experiences of adversity and the spiritual realm.

The contribution of this book is that the African Independent Churches are churches that find a balance between faith healing and indigenous knowledge. The Zion Christian Church, as one of the largest on the continent, is relevant in helping us to understand the intersections of Christianity and indigenous knowledge in the African Independent Churches. This church epitomizes healing that takes from both the Christian faith and indigenous knowledge. Therefore, the African Independent Churches serve as a perfect example of a religious movement that can combine both indigenous knowledge and faith healing. This aspect is important for future studies that seek to understand the African Independent Churches; it would be important to pay attention to the intersections of indigenous knowledge and Christian practices in these churches within the framework of the ritual healing process.

Conclusion

This chapter looked at the findings in the book on the dissociations of traditional African medicine from the ritual healing process in the Zion Christian Churches. The chapter found that the practices of many healing rituals of the Zion Christian Church are distinct from traditional African medicine. In addition, it was important to make a distinction between traditional African medicine and the indigenization of the gospel by the Zion Christian Church and other African Independent Churches. Traditional African medicine is different from indigenization, which is the combination of the indigenous knowledge system and the Christian faith. Both the disconnections with traditional African medicine and the indigenization of the gospel are important in the development of ritual healing theology in the African Independent Churches by using the Zion Christian Church as a case study. This theology is developed through a balance between indigenous knowledge and faith healing within the ritual healing process. This theology makes a distinction between traditional African medicine and faith healing. It is a theology that finds a balance between modern medicine and the indigenous knowledge system and is therefore relevant to an African context. Lastly, this theology places the importance of God as a healer and the faith of patients ahead of the healing rituals.

References

Abrams, A. (2021). *African Goddess Initiation: Sacred Rituals for Self-Love, Prosperity, and Joy*. Hay House.

Adogame, A. (2000). Aiye loja, orun nile: The appropriation of ritual space-time in the cosmology of the Celestial Church of Christ. *Journal of Religion in Africa*, *30*(1), 3–29.

Adogame, A., Adedibu, B. A., Akindolie, A. A., and Olujobi, A. A. (2022). The 'invisible enemy' COVID-19 and the responses of Aladura churches in South West Nigeria. *Theologia Viatorum*, *46*(1), 138.

Akyeampong, E. K., and Gates Jr, H. L. (2012). *Dictionary of African Biography* (Vol. 1). OUP USA.

Anderson, A. (1991). *Moya: The Holy Spirit in an African Context*. University of South Africa Press.

Anderson, A. (1999). The gospel and culture in Pentecostal mission in the Third World. *Missionalia: Southern African Journal of Mission Studies*, *27*, 220–30.

Anderson, A. (1999). The lekganyanes and prophecy in the Zion Christian Church. *Journal of Religion in Africa*, *29*(3), 285–312.

Anderson, A. (2000). *Zion and Pentecost: The Spirituality and Experience of Pentecostal and Zionist/Apostolic Churches in South Africa*. University of South Africa Press.

Anderson, A. (2001). Types and butterflies: African-initiated churches and European typologies. *International Bulletin of Missionary Research*, *25*, 107–13.

Anderson, A. (2018). *Spirit-Filled World: Religious Dis/continuity in African Pentecostalism*. Palgrave Macmillan.

Asamoah-Gyadu, J. K. (2014). Therapeutic strategies in African religions: Health, herbal medicines and indigenous Christian spirituality. *Studies in World Christianity*, *20*(1), 70–90.

Asante, M. K., and Mazama, A. eds. (2009). *Encyclopedia of African Religion* (Vol. 1). Sage.

Auerbach, P. S. (2011). *Wilderness Medicine E-Book: Expert Consult Premium Edition-Enhanced Online Features*. Elsevier Health Sciences.

Austnaberg, H. (2008). *Shepherds and Demons: A Study of Exorcism as Practised and Understood by Shepherds in the Malagasy Lutheran Church*. Peter Lang.

Adams, T. E., Ellis, C., and Jones, S. H. (2017). Autoethnography. In *The International Encyclopedia of Communication Research Methods*, ed. M. Allen, 1–11. Sage Publications.

Bird, S. R. (2010). *The Big Book of Soul: The Ultimate Guide to the African American Spirit*. Hampton Roads Publishing.

Bird, S. R. (2022). *The Healing Power of African-American Spirituality: A Celebration of Ancestor Worship, Herbs and Hoodoo, Ritual and Conjure*. Hampton Roads Publishing.

Bird, S. R. (2024). *The Healing Tree: Botanicals, Remedies, and Rituals from African Folk Traditions*. Red Wheel/Weiser.

Bongmba, E. K. (2015). Studying African Christianity: Future trajectories. In *Routledge Companion to Christianity in Africa*, 555–63. Routledge.

Bowen, G. A. (2009). Document analysis as a qualitative research method. *Qualitative Research Journal*, *9*(2), 27–40.

Braun, V., and Clarke, V. (2006). Using thematic analysis in psychology. *Qualitative Research in Psychology*, *3*(2), 77–101.

Brockman, N. C. (2011). *Encyclopedia of Sacred Places [2 volumes]:[2 volumes]*. Bloomsbury Publishing USA.

Brown, R. M. (2012). *African-Atlantic Cultures and the South Carolina Lowcountry*. Cambridge University Press.

Cabrita, J. (2018). *The People's Zion: Southern Africa, the United States, and a Transatlantic Faith-Healing Movement*. Harvard University Press.

Carrasco, L. N., Zulu, M., and Bukasa, P. K. (2019). Steaming in the fringes; healing rituals in Johannesburg. *International Journal of Complementary and Alternative Medicine*, *12*(2), 59–64.

Census (2001). Primary Tables: Census '96 and 2001 compared (PDF). Pretoria: Statistics South Africa. 2004. 25–8. ISBN 0-621-34320-X. Archived from the original (PDF) on 5 May 2005. Retrieved 1 December 2014.

Chaplain, T. L. M. (1986). The Old Testament and effective evangelism in Africa. *International Review of Mission*, *75*(300), 400–9.

Chiorazzi, A. (2015). The spirituality of Africa. *The Harvard Gazette*, 6.

Chitakure, J. (2017). *African Traditional Religion Encounters Christianity: The Resilience of a Demonized Religion*. Wipf and Stock Publishers.

Chukwuma, Onyekachi G. (2022). Old Testament dietary laws in contemporary African Christian practice. *Verbum et Ecclesia 43*(1), 1–9.

Clarke, P. (2004). *Encyclopedia of New Religious Movements*. Routledge. Constitution of the Zion Christian Church (1946).

Creighton, N. (2024). *Green Witchcraft: Connecting with Nature for Spiritual Growth: Unveil the Magic of the Natural World and Harness the Power of the Earth*. Self-published

Csordas, T. J. (1983). The rhetoric of transformation in ritual healing. *Culture, Medicine and Psychiatry*, *7*(4), 333–75.

Csordas, T. J. (1999). Ritual healing and the politics of identity in contemporary Navajo society. *American Ethnologist*, *26*(1), 3–23.

Daneel, M. L. (1987). *Quest for Belonging: Introduction to a Study of African Independent Churches* (Vol. 17). Mambo Press.

Daneel, M. L. (1991). The liberation of creation: African traditional religious and independent church perspectives. *Missionalia: Southern African Journal of Mission Studies, 19*(2), 99–121.

Daneel, M. L. (2000). *African Initiated Churches in Southern Africa: Protest Movements or Mission Churches?* (No. 33). African Studies Center, Boston University.

Daneel, M. L. (2019). *Zionism and Faith-Healing in Rhodesia: Aspects of African Independent Churches* (Vol. 2). Walter de Gruyter GmbH & Co KG.

Daneel, M. L., and Robert, D. L. eds. (2001). *African Christian Outreach: African Initiated Churches* (Vol. 1). Southern African Missiological Society.

Ephirim-Donkor, A. (2015). *African Personality and Spirituality: The Role of Abosom and Human Essence.* Lexington Books.

Ephirim-Donkor, A. (2016). *African Religion Defined: A Systematic Study of Ancestor Worship among the Akan.* Rowman & Littlefield.

Ephirim-Donkor, A. (2021). *African Spirituality: On Becoming Ancestors.* Rowman & Littlefield.

Etherington, Norman. (1979). The historical sociology of independent churches in south east Africa. *Journal of Religion in Africa, 10*(2), 108–26. https://doi.org/10.1163/157006679X00117

Feierman, S. (1985). Struggles for control: The social roots of health and healing in modern Africa. *African Studies Review, 28*(2–3), 73–147.

Feierman, S., and Janzen, J. M. eds. (1992). *The Social Basis of Health and Healing in Africa* (No. 30). University of California Press.

Field, M. (2022). Decolonizing healing through indigenous ways of knowing. In *Reimagining Science Education in the Anthropocene*, ed. M. F. Wallace, J. Bazzul, M. Higgins and S. Tolbert, 121–34. Springer Nature.

Frey, S. R., and Wood, B. (2000). *Come Shouting to Zion: African American Protestantism in the American South and British Caribbean to 1830.* University of North Carolina Press.

Go, J. ed. (2016). *Postcolonial Sociologies: A Reader.* Emerald Group.

Grant, N. K., and Mansell, D. J. (2008). *A Guidebook to Religious and Spiritual Practices for People Who Work with People.* iUniverse.

Gumede, M. V. (1990). *Traditional Healers: A Medical Practitioner's Perspective.* Johannesburg: Skotaville.

Gumo, S., Gisege, S. O., Raballah, E., and Ouma, C. (2012). Communicating African spirituality through ecology: Challenges and prospects for the 21st century. *Religions, 3*(2), 523–43.

Hanekom, C. (1975). *Krisis en Kultus: Geloofsopvattinge en seremonies binne 'n Swart Kerk*, Academica: Kaapstad en Pretoria.

Harrington, N. (2022). *Living with the Dead.* Oxbow Books.

Hoffmann, D. (2003). *Medical Herbalism: The Science and Practice of Herbal Medicine.* Simon and Schuster.

Horton, R. (1967). African traditional thought and Western science. *Africa, 37*(2), 155–87.

Humbe, B. P. (2023). Vaccination in African Initiated Churches in Zimbabwe: A recipe for church ideological bisection. In *Religion and COVID-19 Vaccination in Zimbabwe*, ed. T. Muyambo, F. Sibanda and E. Chitando, 204–19. Routledge.

Ikwuagwu, O. A. (2006). Initiation in African Traditional Religion: A Systematic Symbolic Analysis, with Special Reference to Aspects of Igbo Religion in Nigeria (Doctoral dissertation, Universität Würzburg).

Jacobs, J. L. (2021). The effects of ritual healing on female victims of abuse: A study of empowerment and transformation. In *Gender and Religion*, ed. W. H. Swatos Jr, 127–41. Routledge.

Janzen, J. M., (1992). *Ngoma: discourses of healing in Central and Southern Africa* (Vol. 34). University of California Press.

Joubert, E., Gelderblom, W. C. A., Louw, A., and de Beer, D. (2008). South African herbal teas: Aspalathus linearis, Cyclopia spp. and Athrixia phylicoides – A review. *Journal of Ethnopharmacology, 119*(3), 376–412.

Katongole, E. M. ed. (2017). *African Theology Today.* Wipf and Stock Publishers.

Kgatle, M. S. (2016). Servant Leadership in Mark 10: 35–45 Applied to African Pentecostal Christianity. PhD thesis, University of Pretoria.

Kgatle, M. S. (2019a). Singing as a therapeutic agent in Pentecostal worship. *Verbum et Ecclesia, 40*(1), 1–7.

Kgatle, S. (2019b). *The Fourth Pentecostal Wave in South Africa: A Critical Engagement.* Routledge.

Kgatle, M. S. (2021). *Pentecostalism and Cultism in South Africa.* Palgrave Macmillan.

Kgatle, M. S. (2023). *Prophecy and Politics in South African Pentecostalism: A Pentecostal Political Theology in Postcolonial Africa.* Springer Nature.

Kgatle, M. S., and Mashau, T. D. (2023). A decolonial perspective on the practice of unveiling tombstones in Pentecostal and charismatic churches in South Africa. *Religions, 14*(3), 288.

Khathide, A. G. (2010). *Hamba Vangeli Elisha: A Portrait of Rev Job Y Chiliza-Pioneer of the African Gospel Church.* Acad SA.

Khorommbi, N. L. (2001). Lutherans and Pentecostals in Mission amongst the Vhavenda: Comparative Study in Missionary Methods. *Unpublished PhD Thesis,* University of South Africa.

Kidwell, M. D. (2014). 'Music therapy and spirituality: How can I keep from singing?', *Music Therapy Perspective 32*(2), 129–35.

Kirmayer, L. J. (1993). Healing and the invention of metaphor: The effectiveness of symbols revisited. *Culture, Medicine and Psychiatry, 17*(2), 161–95.

Koss-Chioino, J. D. (2006a). Spiritual transformation, relation, and radical empathy: Core components of the ritual healing process. *Transcultural Psychiatry, 43*(4), 652–70.

Koss-Chioino, J. D. (2006b). Spiritual transformation, ritual healing, and altruism. *Zygon®, 41*(4), 877–92.

Kruger, M., and Saayman, M. (2016). Understanding the Zion Christian Church (ZCC) pilgrims. *International Journal of Tourism Research, 18*(1), 27–38.

Kumalo, S., and Mujinga, M. (2017). 'Now we know that the enemy is from within': Shembeites and the struggle for control of Isaiah Shembe's Legacy and the church. *Journal for the Study of Religion, 30*(2), 122–53.

Last, M. and Chavunduka, G. L. eds., 1986. *The Professionalisation of African Medicine* (No. 1). Manchester University Press.

Lazar, K. (2005). Why play and sing? The role of folk games and folk songs in everyday life. *Traditiones 34*(1), 191–7.

Lebeloane, L., and Madise, M. (2006). The use of different types of water in the Zion Christian Church. *Studia Historiae Ecclesiasticae, XXXII*(2).

Lekganyane, B. E. (2019a). Ecological sustainability as a topic of redemption within the Theology of the Zion Christian Church. Public Keynote Lecture. *The ZCCMessenger, 105*, 6–10.

Lekganyane, B. E. (2019b). Sermon delivered by his grace, the right reverend Bishop Dr. B. E. Lekganyane on the consecration of the New Year in Zion city Moria, on Sunday 01 September 2019. *The ZCC Messenger, 105*, 13–6.

Lukhaimane, E. K. (1980). The Zion Christian Church of Ignatius (Engenas) Lekganyane, 1924 to 1948: An African Experiment with Christianity (Doctoral dissertation, University of the North).

Maahlamela, T. D. (2017). Sepedi oral poetry with reference to Kiba traditional dance of South Africa. *Dissertation Rhodes University, 20i7.* http://hdl.handle.net/10962/63209.

Magliocco, S. (2010). *Witching Culture: Folklore and Neo-Paganism in America.* University of Pennsylvania Press.

Mahomoodally, M. F. (2013). Traditional medicines in Africa: An appraisal of ten potent African medicinal plants. *Evidence-Based Complementary and Alternative Medicine, 2013*(1), 617459.

Mankga, R. W. (2013). Language Usage in Some Traditional Rituals in Northern Sotho (Doctoral dissertation, University of Limpopo (Turfloop Campus)).

Marks, D. F. (2012). *Overcoming Your Smoking Habit.* Robinson.

Marumo, P. O., and Chakale, M. V. (2018). Understanding African philosophy and African spirituality: Challenges and prospects. *Gender and Behaviour, 16*(2), 11695–704.

Masango, M. J. (2006). African spirituality that shapes the concept of Ubuntu. *Verbum et Ecclesia, 27*(3), 930–43.

Mashabela, J. K. (2017). Healing in a cultural context: The role of healing as a defining character in the growth and popular faith of the Zion Christian Church. *Studia Historiae Ecclesiasticae, 43*(2), 1–14.

Mashabela, J. K. (2023). Africa Independent Churches as Amabandla Omoya and Syncretism in South Africa. *Religions, 14*(11), 1369.

Mbiti, J. S. (1976), Theological impotence and the universality of the Church. In *Mission Trends No. 3,* ed. G. H. Anderson and T. F. Stransky, 6–18. Paulist Press.

Mbiti, J. S. (1990). *African Religions & Philosophy*. Heinemann.

Mbiti, J. S. (1991), *Introduction to African Religion*, 2nd. edn, EAEP.

Mbiti, J. S. (2015). *Introduction to African Religion*. Waveland Press.

McClenon, J. (2004). What is to be done: Evaluating ritual healing theory. In *Proceedings of Presented Papers, The 47th Annual Convention of the Parapsychological Association* (pp. 121–34).

McGuire, M. B., and Kantor, D. (1988). *Ritual Healing in Suburban America*. Rutgers University Press.

Mokgobi, M. G. (2014). Understanding traditional African healing. *African Journal for Physical Health Education, Recreation and Dance, 20*(sup-2), 24–34.

Moripe, S. (1996). The Organisation and Management of the Zion Christian Church (Doctoral Dissertation, Durban Westville).

Moripe, S. (1998). Holiness and taboo in the Zion Christian Church. *Acta Theologica, 18*(1), 1–9.

Morton, B. (2013). The big con: John Alexander Dowie and the spread of Zionist Christianity in Southern Africa Paper. *University of Leiden, African Studies Center, 20*, 1–17.

Morton, B. (2018). *Engenas Lekganyane and the Early ZCC: An Unauthorized History*. PublishDrive.

Mosia, M. J. (2022). *Pandemic Survival Guide: Memory Verses*. Wipf and Stock Publishers.

Mosupyoe, B.Y. (1999). *How Women in the Zion Christian Church of South Africa Mediate Patriarchy and Non-sexism with Their Social Development*. University of California.

Müller, R. (2015). The Zion Christian Church and Global Christianity: Negotiating a tightrope between localisation and globalisation. *Religion, 45*(2), 174–90.

Müller, R. (2016). *African Pilgrimage: Ritual Travel in South Africa's Christianity of Zion*. Routledge.

Mwaura, P. N. (2004). African instituted churches in East Africa. *Studies in World Christianity, 10*(2), 160–84.

Mwaura, P. N. (2007). Religion and leadership: The creation of a just society. *Good governance and development*. In *Toward Quality Leadership in Kenya: Toward Quality Leadership in Kenya*, ed. K. Njogu, 176. African Books Collective.

Mwaura, P. (2014). East African consultation. In *Engaging the World Christian Communities in Contemporary Global Societies*, ed. A. U. Adogame, J. McLean and A. Jeremiah, 211. Regnum Books International.

Mwiti, Salome Gathoni, Nderitu, Joyce W., and Nderitu Wambugu, Simon. (2015). Innovative Christian strategies for confronting syncretic practices in selected Methodist and Pentecostal churches in Abogeta division, Meru County, Kenya. *International Journal of Social Science and Humanities Research 3*(42).

Nel, M. (2005). PL le Roux, Dutch Reformed missionary, Zionist preacher and leader of the Apostolic Faith Mission of South Africa, and the origin of some of the African Independent Churches in Southern Africa. *Dutch Reformed Theological Journal= Nederduitse Gereformeerde Teologiese Tydskrif, 46*(1–2), 200–8.

Nel, M. (2020). T*he Prosperity Gospel in Africa: An African Pentecostal Hermeneutical Consideration*. Wipf and Stock Publishers.

Nthabu, B. Y. (1989). *Meaning and Symbolism in the Zion Christian Church in South Africa*. University of California.

Odoyoye, M. A. (1995). *Daughters of Anowa. African Women and Patriarchy*. Orbis.

Olupona, J. K. (2014). *African Religions: A Very Short Introduction* (Vol. 377). USA: Oxford University Press.

Onwueme, I. C. (2014). *Like a Lily among Thorns: Colonial African Village Child Transitions to Post-Colonial Modernity, and America*. AuthorHouse.

Oosthuizen, G. C. (1992). *The Healer-Prophet in Afro-Christian Churches* (Vol. 3). Brill.

Oosthuizen, G. C. (2000). The African independent churches in South Africa: A history of persecution. *Emory International Law Review, 14*(1), 1089.

Ozili, P. K. (2020). Covid-19 in Africa: Socioeconomic impact, policy response and opportunities, MPRA Paper No. 99617, Posted 17 April 2020, 10:55 UTC, viewed 13 April 2020, from https://mpra.ub.uni-muenchen.de/99617/.

Ozioma, E. O. J., and Chinwe, O. A. N. (2019). Herbal medicines in African traditional medicine. In *Herbal Medicine*, ed. P Builders, 10, 191–214. BoD–Books on Demand.

Rafapa, L. (2013). Popular music in the Zion Christian Church. *Muziki, 10*(1), 19–24.

Rafapa, L. (2018). Distinctive identity in the worship music of the Zion Christian Church within the category of African Initiated Churches. *Muziki, 15*(2), 17–43.

Rakuambo, Z. J., Du Toit, E. S., Soundy, P., and Olivier, J. (2009). Indigenous knowledge system of bush tea from the local people in Venda. *Indilinga African Journal of Indigenous Knowledge Systems, 8*(2), 158–62.

Ramantswana, H. (2018). Prophets praying for, or preying on people's faith: A reflection on prophetic ministry in the South African context. *In die Skriflig, 53*(4), 1–8.

Ranger, Terence. (2007). African Initiated Churches. *Transformation 24*(2), 65–71. https://doi.org/10.1177/026537880702400201.

Reeder, M. (2012). *A Sangoma's Story: The Calling of Elliot Ndlovu*. Penguin Random House South Africa.

Rio, K., MacCarthy, M., and Blanes, R. (2017). *Pentecostalism and Witchcraft: Spiritual Warfare in Africa and Melanesia* (p. 311). Springer Nature.

Sackey, B. M. (2006). *New Directions in Gender and Religion: The Changing Status of Women in African Independent Churches*. Lexington Books.

Sanneh, L., and McClymond, M. eds. (2016). *The Wiley Blackwell Companion to World Christianity*. John Wiley & Sons.

Sax, W. (2014). Ritual healing and mental health in India. *Transcultural Psychiatry, 51*(6), 829–49.

Schoffeleers, M. (1991). Ritual healing and political acquiescence: The case of the Zionist churches in Southern Africa. *Africa, 61*(1), 1–25.

Semenya, D. K., and Letšosa, R. S. (2011). A pastoral investigation of the phrase 'go tloša Setšhila'[traditional purification] as the last phase in the process of bereavement mourning amongst the Basothoase in the process of bereavement mourning amongst the Basotho. *Verbum et Ecclesia, 32*(1), 1–7.

Sered, S. S., and Barnes, L. L. (2007). Teaching healing rituals/ritual healing. In *Teaching Ritual*, ed. C. Bell, 195. Oxford University Press.

Sibam-Twalo, Z., and Ally, Y. (2022). 'I will not Lie to You. The Tokoloshe Exists': Mythical creatures and their influence on mental health amongst a sample of Amaxhosa in the Eastern Cape, South Africa. *Indilinga African Journal of Indigenous Knowledge Systems, 21*(1), 102–18.

Sibanyoni, M. (2020). Zion Christian Church calls off annual Easter pilgrimage until further notice. Viewed 17 March 2020 https://www.sowetanlive.co.za/news/south-africa/2020-03-17-zion-christian-church-calls-off-annual-easter-pilgrimage-until-further-notice/

Sofowora, A. (1996). Research on medicinal plants and traditional medicine in Africa. The *Journal of Alternative and Complementary Medicine, 2*(3), 365–72.

Staub, P. O., Geck, M. S., and Weckerle, C. S. (2011). Incense and ritual plant use in Southwest China: A case study among the Bai in Shaxi. *Journal of Ethnobiology and Ethnomedicine, 7*, 1–16.

Steinbock, R. T. (1982). "Culture, Disease, and Healing". *Studies in Medical Anthropology*, 930–1

Stephenson, B. (2015). *Ritual: A Very Short Introduction*. Oxford University Press.

Stork, J., and Du Toit, C. (2022). Finding ubuntu in the Bible: How the Zion Christian Church in South Africa relates to concepts of ecology in African traditional religions. In *Religious Environmental Activism: Emerging Conflicts and Tensions in Earth Stewardship*, ed. J. Koehrsen, J. Blanc and F. Huber, 198–220. Routledge.

Strohbehn, U. (2016). *The Zionist Churches in Malawi: History-Theology-Anthropology* (No. 17). Mzuni Press.

Sundkler, B. (1961). *Bantu Prophets in South Africa*. Routledge.

Sundkler, B. (1976). *Zulu Zion and Some Swazi Zionists*. Oxford University Press.

Ter Haar, G. (2009). *How God Became African: African Spirituality and Western Secular Thought*. University of Pennsylvania Press.

The ZCC Messenger 5 September 1986.

Turner, E. (1992). *Experiencing Ritual: A New Interpretation of African Healing.* University of Pennsylvania Press.

Ukpong, M. (2015). *Igbo Culture and Gospel: Empirical-Theological Research into Inculturation in Nigeria* (Vol. 7). LIT Verlag Münster.

Van den Bosch-Heij, D. (2013). *Spirit and Healing in Africa: A Reformed Pneumatological Perspective*, 347, UJ Press.

Visser, A. J. (2000). The Kingship of Christ in the Life and Faith of Christians in a Black South African Township: A Missiological Evaluation (Doctoral dissertation, Potchefstroom University for Christian Higher Education).

World Health Organization (2022). Policy response to alcohol consumption and tobacco use during the Covid-19 pandemic in the WHO South-East Asia Region: preparedness for future pandemic events. Snapshot series on alcohol control policies and practice. Brief 7, July 2022. World Health Organization.

White, P. (2015). The concept of diseases and health care in African traditional religion in Ghana. *HTS: Theological Studies, 71*(3), 1–7.

Wouters, J. M. F. (2014). *An Anthropological Study of Healing Practices in African Initiated Churches with Specific Reference to a Zionist Christian Church in Marabastad* (Doctoral dissertation, University of South Africa).

Index

www.ingramcontent.com/pod-product-compliance
Ingram Content Group UK Ltd.
Pitfield, Milton Keynes, MK11 3LW, UK
UKHW020820290926
15470UKWH00003B/1278